COSMETIC
PLASTIC
SURGERY:
A
PATIENT'S
GUIDE

Copyright ©1997 by
Flapartz Press

Canadian Cataloguing in Publication Data

Gelfant, Benjamin, 1954-
Cosmetic plastic surgery: a patient's guide

Includes bibliographical references.
ISBN 0-9682626-0-0

1.Surgery, Plastic. I. Title

RD119.G44 1977   617.9'6   C97-900872-7

Printed in Canada by
Benwell-Atkins

Illustrations by
Hana Kico

Design by
Studio Apropos!

For Zoë and Sophia

BENJAMIN
GELFANT
MD
FRCSC

COSMETIC
PLASTIC
SURGERY
A
PATIENT'S
GUIDE

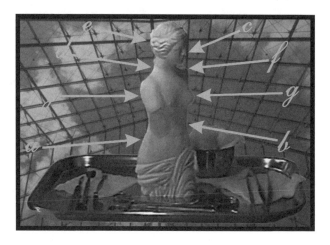

FLAPARTZ
PRESS
1997

ACKNOWLEDGEMENTS

I would like to express my thanks to many people, past and present, who have made this book possible.

Hana and Branislav Klco provided support and artistic input from the time the book was just a loose idea, and were responsible for the design and production. Hana also did the illustrations.

Ira Nadel has been a good friend and a superb editor, and I needed his disciplined, and friendly but scholarly approach.

My devoted and wonderful wife, Barbara, has always been willing to listen, to offer gentle criticism, and help in countless little ways to see the task through to completion. My daughters will both be happy to know they will no longer have to share me with the computer on evenings and weekends.

Joanne Tye, my office manager, has continued to run
a very busy clinical office, so that I would have enough
time to juggle family and clinical responsibilities,
without having to worry about the administrative
matters. My nursing staff have similarly been a joy to
work with.

My thanks also to Lloyd Carlsen, who taught me to be
an esthetic surgeon, to Susan Lowther, who was my
nurse for many years after the start of my practice,
and to the many clinical instructors I had during my
training in plastic surgery.

My father, Harry Gelfant, taught me to be a
professional, in every way, and my mother, Maxine
Gelfant, gave me the interest in reading, writing, and
publishing I needed to want to write this book.

I also wish to express my gratitude to my patients.

TABLE OF CONTENTS

INTRODUCTION

This book has been written to help patients understand the complex and ever changing field of cosmetic surgery, an area of increasing concern to many.

Patients who come for esthetic surgery do not have the imperative of illness putting them in the hands of a doctor for urgent treatment. And while patients often ask, "what do I need, doctor?", there is no need for esthetic surgery, however desirable it may be. Yet there are many, many decisions to be made for each surgical procedure, both in the planning by the patient and the doctor, and in the execution of the operations. The better informed my patient is, the better his or her passage through the pre-operative and post-operative phases.

The many commercially available brochures used by plastic surgery offices to help introduce some concepts of the surgical procedures are often too general. They explain the surgery in a way that gives an overview of the surgery, while omitting the little nuances and differences in surgical approach which might make the difference in why a patient would chose to have surgery with one surgeon or another and the possible complications of surgery.

This book contains as much detail in a book about esthetic surgery as I would usually communicate to my patients in the course of the consultation. But because the nature of the doctor-patient relationship has changed dramatically over the last twenty-five years, in that patients want to, and have a right to, participate in the decision-making process, this book covers the main areas of esthetic surgery in a different way. It has more detail, and may answer many questions but it may also raise others. That would be good. We rarely do an operation the same way for two different patients. Therefore, it is essential for every patient to understand their unique situation, and how I would treat it as their plastic surgeon. This book aims to help explain cosmetic surgery but will not provide the final answers. A proper consultation is the next step.

What follows will serve as a guide to patients seeking information and will provide you with the tools needed to make informed decisions.

The first section of the book will help you to find a plastic surgeon, and know what to expect from a consultation, your financial obligations, the surgeon's obligations, and what is an appropriate facility for the surgery.

In the second section, I will discuss commonly dealt with areas of cosmetic surgery and describe the relevant anatomy so you will find the diagnosis and treatments easier to understand. Previous techniques and current recommendations will be analyzed. I will also consider risks of complications in some detail, so that you will be aware of some of the problems which can occasionally occur. I will also answer some of the most commonly asked questions.

When I consult with my patients for cosmetic surgery, I want them to understand the surgery, the risks, and the likely benefits as much as possible. Trust, in my practice, comes from communication. If this book helps by communicating and making you a knowlegeable patient, it will succeed.

When you have read this book you will be a much better informed patient. But you should not decide on treatment based on what you read in this or any other book alone. This book is intended to be informative, but it is no substitute for a proper consultation with a board certified plastic surgeon about your particular needs. Remember that your relation-ship with your surgeon does not end after you leave the surgical facility, or after the stitches are removed. If you have questions and concerns after your surgery, be sure to discuss them with your surgeon.

THE SEARCH FOR BEAUTY

her beauty made
the bright world dim, and everything beside
seemed like the fleeting image of a shade
                                      Shelley

Whether in women or in men, our favouring of beauty is pervasive. Studies have long shown that society values those who are attractive and beautiful; from infancy onwards, attractive children and, later, handsome adults will be given credit for intelligence disproportionate to their less attractive equals. They also will be viewed as more desirable as friends and are felt to be more honest, trustworthy and romantic than their more common-looking peers. This may be a self-fulfilling prophesy. For example, because 'cuter' babies and children are given more attention, they often grow up with greater confidence. Clearly, beauty, which means pleasing to the senses, has social as well as psychological effects and strongly contributes to our self-esteem and sense of well-being. Not only do standards of beauty determine the relationship an individual will have to her or his body but beauty is often a critical element of romance. As the philosopher Bertrand Russell observed, "on the whole, women tend to love men for their character while men tend to love women for their appearance."

Is this why we spend so much energy in the search for beauty? Perhaps. The art critic John Berger has noted that "soon after we can see, we are aware that we can also be seen." The eye is the fundamental tool of the artist, as the poet William Carlos Williams noted: "Eyes have always stood first in the poet's equipment." This need to be seen is ingrained and implies a desire to be seen at our best, to be recognized and admired. The philosopher Santayana felt "that, for man all nature is a secondary object of sexual passion, and that to this fact the beauty of nature is due." Whatever the cause, books with titles like The Power of Beauty by Nancy Friday, The Beauty Myth by Naomi Wolf or Beauty Bound by Rita Freedman continue to be read and discussed.

Psychologists have studied the role of attractiveness in human evolution, looking for traits said to be associated with the so called "evolutionary success". Certain traits in women, such as smooth skin, smaller noses and ears, and fuller lips, as well as the facial proportions of youth (unlined face, higher cheekbones, narrower cheeks, a slim neck) are associated with vitality, and therefore fertility. These qualities are then perceived as sexually desirable and beautiful. Highly set eyebrows, large smiles, and large pupils, all expressive features, convey sociability. Raised eyebrows often signal interest, and greeting. Individuals whose eyebrows are set relatively high may convey a positive attitude and receive more positive ratings than their low-browed peers. Beautiful traits are felt to be conducive to successful mating and may be more successful, from an evolutionary standpoint.

The reasons why attractiveness is important in society are less important to me as a plastic surgeon than the fact of it being important. Regardless of the time in history, the location in the world, or even the species of plant or animal, form and the aesthetics of form are important. Birds have colourful and attractive plumage (although it is usually the male who wears the flamboyant plumage). Deer and moose have elaborate antlers, flowers display extraordinary arrays of colour and form. In fact it was specifically the dazzling variety and individuality of the plants and animals of the Galapagos which made Darwin realize this was all linked to reproductive biology and evolution. This is so much so that nature's beauty seems to be inherently linked to function, and humans have copied this in endeavors ranging from architecture and engineering, to reconstructive surgery. Historically, humans have adorned themselves with feathers and furs, created elaborate patterns of scars, tattooed their skin and used drugs to enlarge the pupil of the eye, in order to increase their attractiveness.

Some anthropologists have attempted to determine universal measures of attractiveness, but it seems reasonable to view at least some of this to be culturally determined. Aboriginal practices such as lip and ear-lobe stretching, Chinese foot-binding, and tattooing are examples of varying methods of beauty-creating efforts. The changing ideal of beauty as seen in cinema stars through the twentieth century further shows how ideas of beauty shift.

Reconstructive surgery has become more aesthetic as it has become better at achieving function, and the line where reconstruction leaves off and cosmetic surgery begins has become blurred. A well reconstructed hand after a severe injury looks like a normal hand and has the beauty of form which is possessed by a normal hand. Reconstruction of the face for congenital deformity or after cancer surgery results in both near-normal looking and near-normal functioning features if a good result is achieved.

In recent years, cosmetic surgery has become a reasonably safe alternative for those who do not perceive themselves as attractive or beautiful - a satisfying means of achieving a greater measure of attractiveness and beauty.

Some have argued that cosmetic surgery is part of a recent, large-scale effort to control women through enslavement to the worship of unattainable ideals. This argument ignores the biologic forces of attractiveness and the signals which cause us to feel attractiveness and revulsion; it also ignores the cultural biases and indoctrination which each adult woman (and man) encounters. A surprising number of patients come for surgical consultation in their forties and early fifties after being unable to reconcile a feminist ideology with the desire to beautify themselves and stay the inevitable process of aging.

There are certainly a few surgeons who pursue cosmetic surgery for monetary gain alone and with indifference to the health of their patients, who are mostly women. Because the primary role of a doctor in society is to relieve suffering, as a surgeon attempting to improve appearance for a patient and correct deformities when required, I am striving to help that person live more harmoniously in the familial, social, sexual, and even the business environment of everyday life.

Although fashion magazine photographs often seem to promote an ideal which is unrealistic and unhealthy to women, most of my patients are not trying to achieve anything like what is seen in magazines; they merely wish to be normal. And although the definition of normal is partly determined by the surrounding social environment, it is also shaped by the appearance of friends and family. Many times I see patients who want that most controversial of all cosmetic procedures, breast augmentation, partially because their siblings and mothers had larger breasts; similarly, studies have shown repeatedly that patients wanting rhinoplasty (cosmetic nose surgery) simply want to "fit in ". They feel that their noses are very conspicuous. The average cosmetic surgery patient is not wealthy, famous, or terribly vain. I avoid operating on patients who are going to become plastic surgery addicts; they often have deep underlying psychological troubles. The average cosmetic surgery patient is normal in psychological makeup, income and family - and turns to esthetic surgery to enhance an already satisfying life.

THE CONSULTATION

CHOOSING A PLASTIC SURGEON

Warning: not all plastic surgery is done by plastic surgeons.

Prior to the actual surgery, the most significant, and sometimes the most difficult step, is selecting a plastic surgeon. This requires that the patient research the available physicians, telephone the office, make an initial inquiry, and attend the surgeon's office for an initial discussion. Many patients will see two or more surgeons. The contact over the telephone will be first with a receptionist, and much can be gained from that initial telephone discussion.

First, however, how do you decide where to make the initial call?

* family doctor
* "word of mouth": friends and acquaintances who have had surgery
* Yellow Pages
* Magazine, newspaper advertising
* hair stylist, beautician, esthetician, etc.
* Internet

In Canada, most visits to a specialist require a referral from the patient's family doctor because of the structure of the provincial medical plans. Cosmetic surgery is not covered by medical insurance, and, therefore, does not require a referral. The consultation usually takes from thirty minutes to one hour and most plastic surgeons charge a consultation fee. Because the patient pays this fee directly, the decision as to what surgeon he or she sees, or how many consultations to attend, is strictly up to the patient, and does not need to be influenced by the restrictions of the medical insurance plans.

The family doctor, however, may be a useful resource person, and may make a recommendation or give a list of several names. How reliable he or she is depends on a number of factors, including whether his or her personal philosophy is positive or negative towards esthetic surgery. Many patients do not ask their personal physician because they believe, rightly or wrongly, that their doctor disapproves of esthetic surgery as frivolous. The family physician may be less familiar with the current state of esthetic surgery because of the simultaneous movement of esthetic surgery out of the hospital to the private facility and the decreased role of the family doctor in the hospital. But most would be willing and interested to find a good surgeon for their patients. Those who still maintain close contact with their hospital colleagues will be familiar with plastic surgeons doing much traumatic and reconstructive surgery. Some of these plastic surgeons also do excellent esthetic surgery, some do very little. You may need to dig just a little bit deeper to be reasonably certain as to how qualified a surgeon is to deal with your particular problem.

Other sources of information may be useful, or unreliable, depending on the individual situation.

Estheticians and hair stylists, trainers and instructors, may or may not be reliable sources. Certainly, if they see a significant number of clients who have had esthetic surgery, they will be able to comment on such issues as scars, and patient satisfaction. However, all surgeons occasionally encounter complications, and there may be a tendency among lay persons to criticize heavily a surgeon because of one unfortunate case. Similarly, knowing one patient who has had successful surgery and is thrilled is a good reference but it does not mean another patient will have a similar result.

Advertising was long frowned upon, even banned in professional groups, but this began to change in the 1970's. Lawyers argued that advertising was a useful means of professionals informing the public about their services and credentials. Later, court challenges made advertising possible for doctors as well. This has been a mixed blessing. For the patient, advertisements may be informative, but they may also be misleading. My own advertisements, for example, in the Yellow Pages, list the services I offer and my major credentials and certifications.

CREDENTIALS

Because esthetic surgery has not become subject to the same rationing as other aspects of health care, many non-plastic surgeons have been attracted to the relatively "free market". Many persons who are certified as non-plastic-surgery surgeons, non-surgeon medical doctors and even non-M.D.'s (dentists, osteopaths, etc.), are now doing esthetic surgery and patients are faced with difficult and confusing choices.

Certification in plastic surgery means a trained M.D. (who has completed three or more pre-medical school years of university, four years of medical school and certification examinations), and who underwent a further five to seven years residency training, first in all aspects of surgery and then in plastic and reconstructive surgery. He or she would then be recommended by his or her superiors for the privilege of writing a written examination in Plastic and Reconstructive Surgery, administered by the Royal College of Physicians and Surgeons. If this was passed, he or she was then eligible to undergo a further oral examination which, if passed, resulted in certification in Plastic and Reconstructive Surgery. In the U.S.A., the candidate was not allowed to sit for his or her oral exams until a portfolio of personal cases was assembled and submitted to the American Board of Plastic Surgery, which is one of twenty-four specialities accredited by the American Board of Medical Specialities. The certified surgeon may then feel further experience is to his or her benefit and enroll as a fellow in one of the special areas of interest within plastic surgery, such as hand surgery, cranio-maxillofacial surgery (surgery of the jaws, facial bones and skull), burns, or esthetic surgery, usually for a period of six or twelve months.

There are many doctors who have not undergone this training but who have decided to do esthetic surgery. After years of fighting an inter-specialty "turf battle" with their sister specialists in ear, nose and throat surgery, plastic surgeons are beginning to acknowledge that there is no legal way the field of esthetic surgery can be reserved as their exclusive domain, and the argument with ear, nose and throat surgeons (who have aggressively marketed themselves as "facial" plastic surgeons) may finally be subsiding. However, many other specialties, and non-specialists are flooding into the field, including other surgical specialists such as eye surgeons (ophthalmologists) and gynecologists; as well as non-surgical doctors including dermatologists, general practitioners, even dentists. Beware of those who claim to members of the American Board of Cosmetic Surgery or similar such self designated boards not recognized by the American Board of Medical Specialties or the Royal College of Surgeons of Canada. Also ask if the surgeon is board certified and in what field, and ask to see the appropriate certificates. These should be displayed for easy access.

In the end, whether or not a surgeon is right for you for an esthetic surgical procedure depends on many factors, including their qualifications and training, their compassion as a doctor, and their surgical abilities.

To verify a surgeon's credentials, or to get a list of surgeons in the area, one of the best sources is the telephone hotline provided by the Canadian Society for Aesthetic(Cosmetic) Plastic Surgery (1-416-831-7750); the American Society for Plastic and Reconstructive Surgery hotline @1-800-635-0635; or the American Society for Aesthetic Surgery@1-888-272-7711. They will also send information brochures if desired.

The American Society of Plastic & Reconstructive Surgeons can be contacted on the World Wide Web via http://www.plasticsurgery.org. The American Society for Aesthetic Plastic Surgery URL is http://surgery.org

My advice is for a patient to call the above societies to verify whether an individual is or is not a plastic surgeon. You can also ask to see the certificates issued by the Royal College in Canada, or the American Board of Plastic Surgery in the U.S.A.

THE CONSULTATION

Steps in the consultation:

> telephone contact (possible information sent out);
> appointment made
> medical history
> discussion about the specific patient concern
> Examination
> surgeon's assessment, proposed surgical plan, alternatives
> risks of surgery and expected outcome
> photography, paperwork, review of plan and risks, lab tests
> Computer imaging (Optional)

Once you make a telephone call, you should feel, from start to finish, that you are, and will be, handled in a courteous, kind, and professional manner. The telephone reception you receive will be a significant indication of how skilled the surgeon's office is at dealing with your concerns.

The consultation begins from the moment the patient arrives in the office. Some surgeons see all their patients on certain "office days", and you are just as likely to be sitting with a patient recovering from a major accident as you are with an elderly patient recovering from a skin cancer operation or a child with a facial deformity reconstruction. Others prefer to see their esthetic surgery patients on separate days, and, because these consultations are scheduled in a more elective fashion, you may be one of only a few patients or even the only patient in the office at the time.

Most offices will have a medical information form (see appendix) which the receptionist will ask you to fill in as honestly and completely as possible. This information is essential for the doctor to make decisions about the surgery and anaesthesia, as well as your suitability for surgery. Cosmetic surgery is surgery, and should never be regarded as minor. All medications and allergies should be listed as well as previous surgery of all kinds, especially previous esthetic surgery.

The consultation may last from fifteen or twenty minutes to one hour or longer, if necessary. I usually allocate forty-five minutes to an hour for a new consultation with cosmetic surgery patients.

You should not object if the surgeon requests to contact your family doctor for information about your past medical history, and unless you have particular reasons, you should allow him or her access to your past medical records with a prior esthetic surgeon; this information may be invaluable when secondary surgery is being contemplated.

The surgeon will generally want to know the main reason you are seeking advice and why at this time. The more clearly you can express your concerns, the better the surgeon can address them. Do not come to a consultation and ask "Tell me doctor, what can you do for me?" or "what do I need?". However, the surgeon may, if you ask about one specific area, feel it is necessary to comment on something else in order to ensure you are getting the complete picture (such as mentioning a weak chin in the course of discussing the appearance of your nose).

The surgeon will then need to examine you, and this will involve first a general inspection of the areas of concern. Depending on whether this is a facial matter, or involves the body, this may be done with you sitting and fully clothed, or may require you to disrobe partially or completely. This is a matter which requires confidence in the doctor, and you should feel you are being treated courteously and profes- sionally. I offer my patients a gown, and a curtained-off area to change in. A friend or a family member may participate in the consultation. Some doctors, because of the current state of medico-legal affairs, insist on having a female staff member present when they examine women patients.

After a period of discussion, the surgeon will begin the examination with assessment by palpation, by feeling. For the aging face, this involves gentle pushing and pinching to assess excess skin, looseness of the deeper layers, thickness of the fatty tissues, and the underlying muscle anatomy. For the nose, this involves similar feeling of the skin and soft structures, as well as pressing the bones and cartilages to assess their contributions to the shape of the nose; it will also involve looking inside the nose with a light to assess the interior of the nose and its airflow characteristics.

Breast and body surgery require assessment of the body as a whole, and may require a brief period with the gown removed. The surgeon will want to assess the breasts for relative size, feel for lumps, assess the skin quality, and may check nipple sensation, especially if there was previous surgery.

Body contour surgery evaluation requires numerous "pinch tests", in which the skin and fatty layer are assessed for thickness at various points by pinching; however, this should be gentle and not cause significant discomfort.

I frequently use a surgical marking felt pen to demonstrate incisions, mark body contours which are to be treated, and to help patients understand how surgery would be done. The ink is easily wiped off when the consultation ends using alcohol pads.

X - rays and laboratory information, which may be required, are important but of less significance in cosmetic plastic surgery than in many other areas of medicine. Most decision-making is based on information gained verbally from the patient and by the examination.

Once an assessment of the patient as a whole and of the

specific areas of concern is completed, a discussion takes place, including the surgeon's recommendations, and possible treatment alternatives. You should expect a full and frank analysis of the risks of surgery, well in advance of the surgery date. Questions you have should be answered in a direct and professional manner. The surgeon may choose to show you photographs of typical surgical cases. Photographs should be done in properly comparable poses with consistent lighting, angle and distance from the camera, in order to make any conclusions about results. In the computer era we live in, it is possible to retouch digitally images in such a way that they may misrepresent the results, or even make dramatic changes without any surgery at all. Be sure what you are seeing is accurate.

At the time of the initial visit, I usually provide the patient with a written fee quotation. If I feel I have been unable to reach a conclusion about a treatment plan, more time and even future visits may be required. I usually see my patients at least twice prior to the surgery day, completing the necessary paperwork, answering residual questions, documenting the case photographically, and ordering the necessary lab work at a second visit. If there are relevant medical conditions, I can discuss the patient with her or his family doctor in the interim. This also allows the patient to come to a better understanding of the surgery and the risks.

WHAT ABOUT COMPUTER IMAGING?

As far as I know, I was the first surgeon in Western Canada to use a computer to help demonstrate the possibilites of surgery to patients prior to the operation. A digital camera is used to "capture" an image onto the computer screen, and the computer is then used to simulate the effects of surgery by drawing changes to the patient image. It is not a method of simulating surgery, but simply allows me to show what I hope will be the expected outcome of the operation. Thus the "after" image is more dependent on my skill as a computer artist than on my skill as a surgeon. Moreover, it is a two-dimensional tool, and we are trying to discuss three dimensional areas of concern. So it is more useful, for example, in showing the effects of nose or chin surgery in profile (which is mainly two dimensional) than in a full frontal view.

The major concern expressed at the time the computer became available for imaging was that it could be used as a tool to help sell an operation. When I was interviewed for the daily newspaper and for television, I tried to emphasize that I was using it to help educate patients and clarify the possible limits and benefits of surgery.

Although computer imaging has educational value, it is also a source of confusion rather than clarification. Occasionally, it helps me to realize that a patient has unrealistic expectations of surgery, but I no longer make it part of my routine consultation and use it less and less as time goes on. Most of what needs to be communicated can be done in more traditional ways for patients who have realistic expectations and reasonable insight. A recent article in *Allure* magazine which surveyed several well known esthetic plastic surgeons came to similar conclusions.

PAYMENT

The standard in plastic surgery over the years has been for full payment in advance. Most reputable plastic surgical offices continue with this policy, and require sufficient time for personal cheques to clear (usually one or two weeks) in advance of the surgery. Many now also accept the major credit cards for payment.

Financing of surgery may be offered through the surgeon's office, through third party credit agencies. This is generally a promotional device which is costly to the patient. I do not encourage financing the cost of cosmetic surgery because, if patients are good credit risks, the chartered banks will make consumer loans, at interest rates far lower than patients would receive through the surgeons offices. You are far better off to save the money in a savings account or in an interest bearing certificate throught the bank than to pay a credit agency the high (18 to 24% or higher) interest rates.

My office policy is for a deposit at the time of booking surgery, with the balance due one week prior to the operation. We accept cash, certified cheque, money order, and major credit cards.

SECONDARY SURGERY

When cosmetic surgery results in a less than optimal outcome, a secondary surgical procedure may be required. If you still have a good relationship with your surgeon, it is best to continue with him or her. Most surgeons will not charge, in most cases, a professional fee for secondary surgery on their own patients. However, the cost of the operating room and anaesthesia may be considered the patient's responsibility. Clarify this with your doctor before surgery.

If you seek secondary surgery from another surgeon, he or she will, in general, charge a full professional fee, plus operating room and anaesthesia costs. Fees for secondary surgery may even be somewhat higher because re-operation may be more difficult than the initial surgery.

WHAT IF THERE ARE COMPLICATIONS?

In general, the costs for care of complications are included in the initial fees. Currently, hospitalization for care of complications, although rare, is covered under the provincial medical insurance plans of most Canadian provinces. In the U.S.A., this is not so, and responsibility for after care hospitalization should be known by you, as a patient, prior to undergoing surgery in the United States.

WHERE IS THE SURGERY DONE?

Ten years ago most esthetic surgery was done in public hospitals. But esthetic surgery patients at the public hospitals were increasingly given lower priority both by the administration, resulting in difficulties in scheduling, and by the hospital staff, who were busy dealing with increasingly sicker patients. Today, most surgery is done on an outpatient basis, and nearly all esthetic surgery is done in private clinics. Nonhospital facilities have grown in popularity because of reduced cost, more efficient service, and specialization in the care of the ambulatory patient.

With this move away from the hospital, came a new need for standards. In Canada, the Canadian Association for Accreditation of Ambulatory Surgical Facilities and in the U.S.A., the American Association for Accreditation of Ambulatory Plastic Surgical Facilities, were formed to ensure quality and patient safety. In British Columbia, the College of Physicians and Surgeons began an accreditation programme in the late 1980's which continues. In the mid-1990's, similar accreditation was begun in California, but most states and provinces still do not have such standards, so in other locations the patient should check to ensure the facility is certified by the CAAASPF, or, in the USA, by the the AAAAPSF, the AAAHC, or the JCAHQ.

Regardless of whether the surgery is done under general anaesthesia (the patient completely unaware of the surroundings) or local anesthesia with sedation ("twilight" anaesthesia, in which the patient is less aware of the surroundings but able to respond to spoken orders), the patient will be asked to eat and drink nothing except approved medications, for several hours prior to surgery (usually nothing to eat or drink after midnight the night before). In many cases of twilight anaesthesia, the sedation is given by nurses under the surgeon's direction and no anesthesiologist is present. Whenever a general anaesthetic is given, an anaesthetist is present, although in the U.S.A., certified nursing anesthesia technicians may be used. All patients need to spend at least the first few hours, preferably the first night, in the care of a responsible adult. I usually see patients the first or second working day after surgery and check carefully for any problems, discuss how the patient is feeling, and review any concerns.

RESTORING THE FACE

SKIN CARE AND SCARS

There is a bewildering array of skin and hair care products confronting men and women in magazine and television advertising, at cosmetic counters and in pharmacies. The production and sales of these products is a huge industry. There are many claims made that these products can make a significant difference in skin tone, and appearance; that they can restore youth, eliminate cellulite, reduce or eliminate bags under the eyes.

Most of the claims made about these products are simply not true.

The single most important thing you can do for your skin is to wear a sun block every day. All ultraviolet rays damage the skin. Tanning is a treatment for animal skins which makes leather tough, coloured, and suitable for uses such as for clothing, saddles, and gloves. Sun-tanning will eventually make your skin thickened and tough with irregular brown areas, wrinkles, and dilated blood vessels. It may also develop skin cancers which will need to be removed surgically (basal cell or squamous cell) leaving small or extensive scars, or may even kill you (melanoma). A good sun block will prevent damage from the full range of UVA and UVB. You should apply it to all normally exposed areas of the face, neck and hands every morning. Tanning beds should not be used. When you are involved in activities that expose you to especially high doses of solar radiation, such as skiing or water sports, a complete block in the most vulnerable areas, reinforced throughout the day, is essential. It is incredibly easy to suffer a second degree radiation burn, with blistering, and a dramatically increased risk of skin cancer while spring skiing.

Treatment with Tretinoin (Vitamin A acid) daily, for a prolonged period, in the right dose, will improve the skin by repairing some of the old damage. It is applied every night and will result in more even skin texture and pigmentation. Small wrinkles will improve.

Wrinkles are caused by environmental damage, mainly radiation from the sun. This is cumulative, meaning that the total dose you have received over your lifetime determines how much damage has been done. If you tanned heavily as a child and teen, that damage is still present and it is especially important to avoid adding insult to injury by continuing to lie in the sun or burning when at a high altitude when spring skiing.

Wrinkles are not caused by dry skin. Moisturizers do not prevent or treat wrinkles. Creams do not feed the skin. Nutrients come to the skin the same way they do to other parts of the body, via the blood stream. Pores do not open and close and breathe. All a moisturizer can do is reduce water evaporation from the skin surface. A water based emollient that does not block pores is all you need to reduce moisture loss. If you smoke, quit. Smoke is as damaging to the skin as it is to other parts of the body. If you smell like smoke, the appearance of your skin won't matter, and non-smokers can always smell a smoker.

In the winter, expect the skin on your body to be dry. Your legs and torso have far fewer oil glands than your face, so are more likely to be dry. Dry skin itches because the main function of skin is as a barrier to the outside world, and dry skin is a less effective barrier. Soap, water and heat will more easily irritate the small nerve endings in the skin. Frequent showers and chemicals in deodorant soaps will only make matters worse. Relatively moist air from outside becomes much less saturated as it is heated by our furnaces to a room temperature, and relative humidity drops. Try to humidify your home to the right level, about 50%, (this is more a factor in the centre of the continent than on the coast, but relative humidity can drop profoundly there as well). Use a simple moisturizer after your shower, while your skin is still damp.

Wash hair with a gentle shampoo every day or two and rinse thoroughly because the shampoo really just frees the dirt and oils from the hair shaft, allowing it to be carried in water. Rinsing thoroughly ensures it is carried away. And shampoo can't do anything more to the hair than help clean it. After that, dress your hair with a light protein gloss or gel type of preparation.

Nails are made of keratin protein and reflect your nutritional status and general health. Proper nutrition, good general health, and gentle care to the nails is the secret to good nails. Do not cut cuticles or push them back. This will only inflame the nail fold, causing it to crack and weaken the nail. Do not use a hard instrument to clean under the nail. Use soap and a nail brush. Every night apply a moisturizer to your nails to reduce evaporation of water.

OTHER TREATMENTS

COLLAGEN

Collagen in skin care products is of absolutely no value. As a large protein molecule, it cannot penetrate through the upper layers of the skin.

Purified collagen protein has been injected into fine and medium wrinkles for about twenty years. A simple office visit is required and the injection takes only a few minutes. A skin test for allergy to the collagen is absolutely required, prior to treatments. It takes several days to see the results of the test, and many doctors feel a second skin test is worthwhile, to prevent allergic reactions to the injected collagen. Collagen treatments are moderately effective but the effects are relatively transient, lasting only three to six months.

I do not use injectable collagen to fill wrinkles and fine lines of the face. It is certainly not a "replacement therapy" as described by the advertisements promoting it. It is made from animal collagen, and is broken down in human skin once injected. In fact your own collagen is in a balance, being constantly made and broken down.

FAT INJECTIONS

Fat injections have limited benefit in the treatment of fine and medium wrinkles, but recent work has shown that part of aging is the gradual loss of fat from the face and therefore the fullness of the face. In a short operation, lasting less than an hour, fat, is injected where it is needed in the face, filling out contours and plumping up the skin. It is taken by liposuction from another part of the body.

BOTOX

A relatively new therapy being used for wrinkles of the brows and around the eyes is Botox, made from the same toxin which causes botulism poisoning, but used in much lower doses. This has been used successfully for years to "fine tune" the results of eye squint surgery, and has recently been applied for cosmetic uses. Injection results in temporary (three to six months) paralysis of the injected muscles, and it is usually used for frown lines and crows foot lines. However, it has no effect on longstanding established wrinkles where the skin has been deeply creased.

SCARS

All surgical procedures result in scars. One of the main skills of plastic surgeons is controlling scar formation. We do this by carefully choosing incision location and pattern, by gently handling the skin with fine, specialized instruments, and by the skillful and careful repair of surgically or traumatically created incisions and wounds.

The development of "minimal incision", or endoscopic surgery, is a significant advance in reducing scars for some operations.

Much of how you will form scars, however, depends on the location of the incision, and your racial and genetic pre-disposition to scarring. People with black African and yellow Asian skin are especially prone to excess scarring, and incisions must be very carefully planned.

Normal scar formation develops according to a rough schedule. During the first few weeks, the scar develops some strength. It usually looks a little pink when the stitches are removed, but is flat. From three to six weeks, it becomes thicker and often redder, as it gains collagen protein, and it looks its worst during this phase. Then maturation begins, and this may take from six to eighteen months, or even longer. During this phase the scar continues to get stronger but gradually flattens, softens, and becomes pale.

Location plays a key role in the outcome. Incisions in the upper eyelids, the lips, the groin, and the armpits are especially good, while incisions in the centre of the chest, upper back and the upper outer arm are particularly prone to bad scars. The face, in general, tends to form good scars, if they are properly planned.

Unsatisfactory scars are either thicker, wider, depressed or raised, uneven, or running in a different direction than the normal skin lines.

Keloids are scars which are very thick, angry looking, red to purple, and continue to grow beyond the borders of the original wound or incision. For example, I occasionally see patients with large masses of scar on the chest from minor acne pustules, and on the arm from vaccinations.

Hypertrophic scars, on the other hand, are scars which have become thickened during the normal healing period, but do not go beyond the original wound edge. They usually settle somewhat, over a longer period than the time needed for a normal scar.

There are many misconceptions about what can be done about scars, and when things should be done. Generally, no surgery should be done to revise, or attempt improvement of the scar, until maturation has occurred. Revision is generally done to even out the level of a scar, improve the orientation relative to the normal skin lines, or narrow it.

Keloids and hypertrophic scars can be difficult to treat. Patience is usually the best treatment for thickened but non-keloid scars. Vitamin E and Aloe Vera extract may make the scar look better during the maturation phase, but studies have not shown that they affect the final result. Vitamin E may retard healing if it is used during the early post-operative period (three weeks). Many other drugs and agents have been and are being investigated but none has proved to be better than time.

Injection of thick scars or keloids with cortisone-like drugs may be helpful in many cases, but this has some side effects and should not be used for scars that are only somewhat thick during normal wound maturation. Pressure has been used for many years for burn scars, and recently has been combined with silicone sheeting laid directly on the scar. Pressure is applied by a variety of means, usually by the use of custom elasticized garments, worn twenty-three or more hours per day for months. Used alone or along with pressure, silicone sheeting has shown some success, and some surgeons now advise it routinely for certain incisions, such as breast lifts and reductions, and for tummy tuck incisions. It must be used twenty-three hours daily as well.

In extreme cases, keloids have been treated with low dose radiation therapy, combined with the other methods described above, but with variable success.

It is unusual to have keloids result from surgery for people with light skin colour, and keloids are rare in cosmetic surgery in general. The location of incisions is carefully and electively chosen, careful technique is used, and most people who may be susceptible to keloids can be warned in advance.

THE FACELIFT: REJUVENATIVE FACIAL SURGERY

The facelift has changed dramatically over the past twenty years. In this chapter I will attempt to explain these changes, how we make alterations both to the skin and the deeper structures to effectively restore more youthful contours.

* Facelift
* Forehead lift
* Blepharoplasty, or eyelid plasty

As a patient considering rejuvenative or restorative surgery of the face, you probably have certain concerns which you consider to be of the greatest importance to you.

The most common areas of concern to patients are:
* loss of a youthful appearing neck
* development of jowls
* deep folds or creases running from the nose past the corners of the mouth, to the chin
* "bags" under the eyes
* excess skin or "hooding" above the eyes
* frown and worry lines above the nose and in the forehead

Rejuvenative surgery now addresses each of these areas in a very specific fashion.

HISTORY

THE FACELIFT

Traditionally, a facelift was performed from the temple around the ears and into the neck using incisions that were relatively visible and only through the skin. Through these incisions, the surgeon operated under the skin for a relatively short distance under the cheeks and then pulled the skin as tight as he dared in an attempt to lift the sagging jowls and cheeks. This skin only operation left many patients with a "wind blown" appearance and unnatural shape to the mouth and the corners of the eyes and was totally ineffective at treating the changes of the neck and jawline. Its effects were relatively short-lived.

In the mid 1970's, after the prompting of surgeons outside of North America, some Canadian and American surgeons began dealing with the thin muscle layer under the skin in the neck and by means of stitching it backwards, or by repositioning it and by removing the excess fat under the chin, they were able to create a more youthful and appealing chin, neck angle and jawline.

About the same time, a Swedish surgeon, Tord Skoog, demonstrated that this muscle layer, which appeared to end at the jawline, actually extended upwards into the cheek right to the cheek bone as a thin but very strong membrane. If this was lifted along with the skin of the face without going just under the skin, Skoog showed, the face could be restored in a much safer and more effective fashion.

Like many good ideas, however, the significance of this was lost on most practising surgeons since it was a revolutionary and very dramatic change from the normal, and because it required entering into areas of anatomy which were poorly understood and were, therefore, intimidating. It has taken twenty years for a more gradual evolution of his ideas to gain widespread acceptance. The operation is considerably more difficult and takes longer to perform but the results are immeasurably greater.

In the interim, a less extensive operation on this layer was gradually accepted as a better way of performing a facelift than the simple skin-only operation. With the advent of liposuction in the 1980's, removal of fat become a common-place procedure both from under the chin where it still remains of considerable use, but also in the cheeks and along the jawline and especially in the area of the nasolabial folds, those deep furrows running down from the nose to the corner of the mouth onto the jowls.

Suddenly, in the late 1980's, certain surgeons in the United States popularized a Skoog-like operation, which had been performed regularly by certain surgeons in Quebec ever since it was described in the 1970's. When finally discovered by the American print and the electronic media, this "deep plane" operation for fat pad repositioning procedure suddenly caught on, and rapidly became the procedure of choice for surgeons who, like their patients, have been frustrated by the limitation of earlier procedures. Instead of suctioning away or cutting away fat from areas where it was felt to be excessive; instead of drawing the skin tightly and hoping this would reposition the underlying structures; and instead of suffering the unnatural pull of the tight membranes when it has not been completely freed, surgeons are now able to lift the skin and the underlying fat pads into a more youthful position and hold them in position by working with the relatively inelastic deep layer, and yet still not rely on extreme tension on the skin to maintain the results. Where it was once felt necessary to remove malpositioned fat pads, we now feel that these fat pads are a sign of youth when properly positioned over the cheek bones and high on the jawline. Similarly, the platysma muscle is now freed from its surrounding attachments and stitched together in the midline under the chin, while also being angled backwards and held with stitches from the back.

THE EYELID PLASTY
BLEPHAROPLASTY

"The eyes are the windows of the soul", an old proverb says.

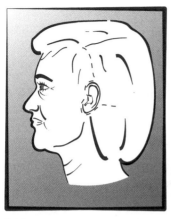

1a)

A facelift primarily addresses sagging of cheeks, jowls, and neck. Incisions are made on each side from inside the hair at the temples, along the ear, and into the scalp behind the ear, as well as under the chin. The exact design varies from patient to patient and from surgeon to surgeon.

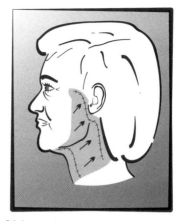

1b)

The deep layers (SMAS and Platysma) are tightened in the neck and in front of the ear.

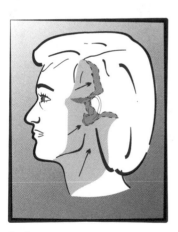

1c)

Tightening of the skin and fat pads then follows.

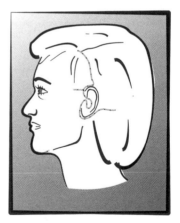

1d)

The result is more youthful appearance without appearing overdone or overtightened. Incisions are concealed as much as possible.

Of all facial rejuvenative procedures, the blepharoplasty is the most commonly performed and has a very substantial benefit compared to the extent of the surgery.

With age, the eyes may take on a tired or fatigued look due to several factors. These may not be related to age and are very commonly associated with your family background but are often interpreted as signs of age. The upper eyelids may develop considerable redundant skin, so much so that it

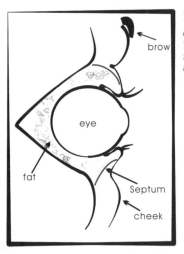

2a)

Cross section of eye and lid. The eye rests in a cushion of fat. This is held back by a thin retaining wall, the septum.

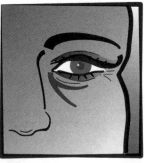

2b)

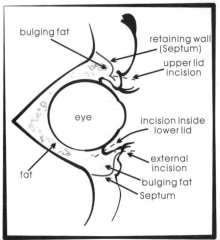

2c)

The retaining wall, or septum, may sag, resulting in "bags" under the eye, and a fatigued appearance. The fat is typically seen in two areas of the upper lids and three in the lower lids. Excess skin may develop in the upper or lower lids.

may actually hang completely over the eyelids and rest on the eyelashes and, in extreme circumstances, may cause some obstruction to vision towards the periphery of your visual field. If this extreme is reached, your medical insurance may cover part or all of the cost.

In order to explain what goes on under the skin, we have to consider some of the anatomy of the eye. The eye sits within the bones of the face floating in a cushion of fat cells. Under normal circumstances, this fat is held in place by a strong but thin membrane or wall which runs from the eyelid

2d)

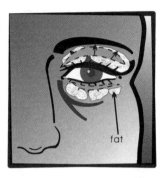

Incisions follow the natural contour lines in the upper and lower lids to give access to skin and protruding fat.

fat

down to the rim of the cheek bone in the lower eyelid and from the upper eyelid up to the brow. In some individuals who are predisposed, this wall gradually or suddenly weakens and the fat begins to bulge into the skin of the eyelids both in the lower and in the upper eyelids. When we see bags under the eyes, this is merely the fat bulging into the skin causing a convexity below the natural border of the eyelid. This is often also seen just above the inner corner of the eye in the upper eyelid.

In performing an eyelid plasty or blepharoplasty, the surgeon trims the excess skin from the upper eyelid and approaches this bulging fat by splitting the membrane, then trims the fat and carefully cauterizes any tiny blood vessels which would otherwise cause bleeding, allows the fat to return to its place and closes the incision with some fine stitches. In the lower eyelid, if there is excess skin, this is trimmed via an incision immediately under the eyelashes which in time becomes very difficult to see. It is uncommon to have a lot of excess skin to the lower eyelids and any attempt to lift the lower eyelid by means of trimming skin may result in the eyelid being pulled downwards and outwards creating a very unsatisfactory appearance. Thus, the surgeon should always be extremely cautious about removing skin from the lower eyelids.

A more recent technique of lower lid blepharoplasty involves removing the lower lid fat from an incision on the inside of the lower lid, leaving no external scar, or just a small scar in

2e)

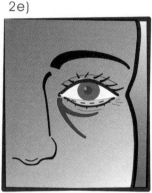

The lower lid fat can also be approached via an incision inside the lid, leaving no external scar and requiring no stitches.

2f)

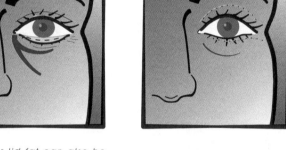

Surgery results in more youthful, rested appearance, with invisible or nearly invisible scars.

the outer corner. If skin tightening is felt to be necessary, this can be done either with a skin-only removal on the outside of the lid, or, can be attempted with one of the new generation of pulsed lasers, which create a very superficial peeling of the skin. When this heals, it does so with some tightening of the skin and with reduction of wrinkles.

Some surgeons now believe that excess removal of fat may lead to a rather hollow and operated look in later years. Most recently, new techniques involving the traditional external incision but with repair and repositioning of the fat pockets, have been developing. The weak wall is repaired and the fat is partially removed with the remainder put back into position.

The choice of what technique is applicable will depend on your own anatomy and the surgeon's preference and experience.

FOREHEAD, OR BROW LIFTS

It is also possible to confuse the brow skin with skin of the upper eyelids. If there is great excess to the brows, the skin of the brow will fall into the region of the eyelids and this is not alleviated by an upper eyelid plasty, only by a forehead and browlift. The facial features treatable by forehead lifting are:
* "hooding" of the upper eyelids
* chronic angry or sad expression
* deep worry or frown lines

The facelift, as it has been traditionally known, is a proce-dure on the cheeks, temple and neck but in modern usage the concept of a complete facelift has to also involve the restoration of the entire face and this also refers to the eyelids and the forehead. When discussing a facelift with your surgeon, a definition of terms is necessary. I refer to a facelift as involving the traditional areas of the cheeks and neck; a forehead lift is an adjunct to this. A traditional

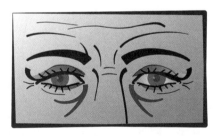

3a)

Pre-operatively, patients for forehead lift may have an angry, sad, or tired expression; hooding of the outer eyes; low brow position; or deep frown lines.

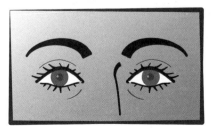

3b)

Post-operatively, the brows are in more pleasing position, hooding and frown lines are reduced, and the forehead is smoother.

Forehead lift

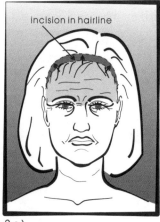

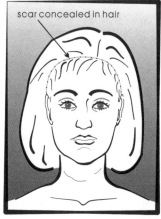

3c)
In an open forehead lift, an incision in or at the hairline is used to approach the brow and frown muscles.

3d)
The resulting scar is usually well concealed within the hair.

Endoscopic forehead lift

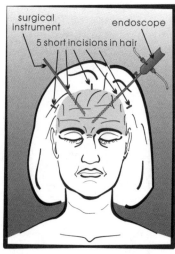

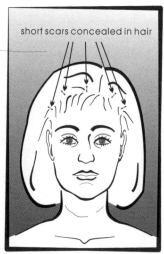

3e)
In an endoscopic forehead lift, several small incisions within the scalp are used. The telescope allows the surgeon to see under the surface, modify the frown muscles, and lift the brow without a long incision.

3f)
The resulting small scars heal rapidly and are well concealed.

forehead lift involves the extension of the facelift from the temple on one side to the temple on the other side by a route either at the edge of hairline in the forehead, or back in the scalp, depending on the shape of your hairline and how high your forehead is.

Recently, the forehead lift has been done via very small incisions using the endoscope, the surgical telescope-like device that has successfully reduced knee surgery scars from long unsightly incisions to much smaller puncture sites. In the forehead lift this offers the advantage of reducing the incision from one which runs from ear to ear across the top of the head, to several very short incisions. The aims of this operation are threefold: to reduce the sagging of the brow,(thus it is often also known as a browlift); to reduce the action of the frown muscles at the top of the nose and between the eyes; and to reduce the frown lines running horizontally across the forehead, if these are a significant feature. In addition, the operation may also give some reduction to the expression lines running from the corners of the eyes [crowfoot lines] and will often contribute to the lift in the upper cheek.

Compared to the cheek and necklift procedure, the forehead lift is relatively straightforward in that the anatomical structures are considerably simpler. In this procedure, the surgeon usually gets under the frown muscles and brow, frees the entire area from its tight attachments along the edge of the bony brow, modifies the muscles so their action produces a more youthful appearance, and lifts the entire forehead into a more youthful position. The small incisions used are easily concealed in the scalp, and recovery is quite rapid, usually about one week before returning to regular activity.

In my practice, approximately 75% of patients undergoing a facelift also have a forehead lift either simultaneously or shortly thereafter, and since the advent of the endoscope, forehead lifts alone or with some eyelid surgery has become much more common, and is often done in younger patients.

SELECTION OF SURGERY

The greatest decision that you need to make is whether the operation will be helpful for you.

If you are expecting a transforming miracle from surgery, you will likely be disappointed. The degree of improvement will be determined by such factors as your age, heredity, the bony architecture of your face and various individual characteristics of your skin and underlying structures. Personal habits such as alcohol intake, your personal nutrition and smoking are important. I have personally chosen not to operate on patients who actively smoke because the rate of serious complications is so vastly increased. One major study has pointed out that the risk of losing a significant area of skin due to poor oxygen supply with a facelift is increased 1500% in active smokers. Surgery is not an exact science and because some of the factors in producing the final result are not entirely within control of either the surgeon or the patient, it is impossible to guarantee results. To further complicate matters by smoking is to add greatly to the risks.

Emotional stability is also one of the most important factors to be established before any esthetic surgery is undertaken. It is vital that you have emotional support in the early days after surgery from friends or family members. If you are having an operation done despite all the protestations of your closest friends or relatives, you will feel very much alone in the early post operative period. This, combined with a very common feeling of letdown in this early period, may make the transition period difficult. There are potential side effects and risks associated with the surgery and should any of these occur in the absence of a positive attitude and emotional support, overcoming them is made significantly more difficult.

There are certain things that we can do in order to try to minimize the risks of post operative complications and these include the avoidance of smoking, encouraging good nutrition and the avoidance of vitamin E and aspirin in the final three weeks prior to surgery as these may seriously contribute to the risk of bleeding. All surgery on the skin leaves scars and despite what you may have heard, all surgical scars are permanent, although they may be planned to be in relatively inconspicuous locations and will gradually fade to become pale and soft. One of the tasks of the surgeon is to plan the incisions so that scars are found in natural lines in the face and eyelids where they are least noticeable and more easily camouflaged.

RISKS OF SURGERY

These include bleeding, infection, injury to sensory or motor nerves, delayed healing, and dissatisfaction with the surgical result.

COMPLICATIONS OF FACELIFT AND FOREHEAD LIFTS

Bleeding, the most common serious complication which occurs in facelifts, is reported to occur in 2-6% of patients, and is more common in men than women. Because a space has been developed under the skin so the fabric (the skin and soft tissues) can be re-draped over the underlying structures, if bleeding under the surface starts in the post - op period, it can accumulate as a large clot, and can put pressure on the skin, thereby causing pain, poor nutrition to the skin, and in severe cases, difficulty breathing. As soon as it is recognized, the surgeon will arrange to remove the clot and stop the bleeding, which usually requires a trip back to the operating room. With proper treatment, a hematoma, as this is known, leaves no permanent effects.

Infection in facelifts is unusual. When it occurs, it is usually mild, and usually easily treated. As with any major surgical procedure, the potential for serious infection exists, but major infection requiring hospitalization and intensive treatment is rare.

Nerve injuries occur only rarely in facelifts. They most

commonly involve a sensory nerve (one which gives feeling,) of the lower ear, or to skin behind the ear. More rarely, a motor nerve, one which causes muscles to move, can be injured. This occurs in less than 1% of facelifts. The most commonly involved muscle is the forehead muscle which raises the brow and causes horizontal frown lines. Less common is one of the small muscles at the the corner of the mouth. Motor nerve injuries are almost always temporary and recovery is almost always complete.

COMPLICATIONS RELATING TO EYELID PLASTY

This can also include infection and bleeding, as with any surgical procedure. Serious bleeding is rare, but if there is severe and increasing pain after surgery, especially on one side, this may indicate ongoing bleeding and the formation of a clot, which may put pressure on the eye. If left untreated, this can lead to loss of vision on that side(an extremely rare circumstance). Sudden increasing pain and swelling should be brought to your doctor's attention immediately, so that, if necessary, measures can be taken to reduce pressure and control bleeding. As with many other types of surgery, but especially with the eyes, the risk of this occurring can be reduced by prior recognition and treatment of high blood pressure, the avoidance of drugs which can promote bleeding such as aspirin or other drugs in the same family, and proper rest and iced compresses in the post-operative period.

Changes to the shape of the eyes can occur and current innovations in techniques are aiming to minimize the risk of this as much as possible. In the past, it was not uncommon for patients to complain that there had been a subtle change in the dimensions of the eye, with the eye appearing more rounded and with a little or more white showing beneath the coloured part (iris) of the eye. Worse, in the occasional patient, the lower lid blepharoplasty resulted in a pulling down of the lower lid, with consequent drying and irritation of the eye. While this situation (ectropion) usually resolves spontaneously with time, it is annoying and disruptive to patient's routine, and sometimes needs to be treated with corrective surgery.

If you have pre-existent problems with the health of your eyes, these may be worsened by blepharoplasty. For this reason, I routinely ask that my patients undergoing blepharoplasty have an eye examination by an eye specialist, during which tear secretion and quality, vision, eyeball pressure, and the retina are examined. Occasional patients have early signs of glaucoma or other diseases, without any symptoms; dryness is relatively common.

DISSATISFACTION WITH THE SURGICAL RESULT

This can stem from two factors. The first is unrealistic expectations on the patient's part. It is important for the surgeon to try to appreciate the patient's concerns during consultation, and excellent communication needs to be established. You should feel comfortable that you can express your concerns to the surgeon, that he or she understands them, and that you will be able to have ongoing communication with your surgeon. Your aims, and the surgeon's aims, should be the same, or what the surgeon may feel is a good surgical result may not be what satisfies you.

The other source of dissatisfaction is a less than optimal surgical result. Again, surgery is an inexact science, and no two patients will respond to a procedure in the same way. For this reason, each patient must be dealt with in an individualized fashion. Even today, with all the techniques, knowledge, and technology we possess, there is no perfect operation, although results are far better than they were even a few years ago. A surgeon with experience will tell you there often are compromises, and that results of surgery evolve to a finished point over many months. Often, patience will reward you with an ultimately satisfying result.

SKIN RESURFACING

Most patients seeking advice from a plastic surgeon about aging wish as complete a restoration of youthful qualities as possible. The focus of plastic surgery has traditionally been on those changes of the structures of the face which can be treated surgically, and this has generally meant dealing with large changes visible from a distance; these, as mentioned in the chapter on facial rejuvenative surgery, include the loss of a defined jawline, or the development of jowls.

Patients, on the other hand, have always been concerned with finer details. Originally, they wanted the facelift and eyelid operations to eliminate wrinkles - wrinkles around the mouth, the eyes, in the cheeks, and even in the neck. It became obvious that the operations could not do these things. As the operations became better and better at smoothing deep folds and sagging deeper tissues, it became clear that other means were needed to smooth the fine wrinkles of the skin.

Another group of patients seeking help with the skin surface are those with extensive irregularities, including pits and scars resulting from acne. Many of these patients have been treated in the past by dermabrasion, with variable results.

ANATOMY

Wrinkles are usually not the result of natural aging and drying of the skin; they are caused by radiation and chemical damage. The radiation comes mainly in the form of harmful sun damage, and chemical injury is most

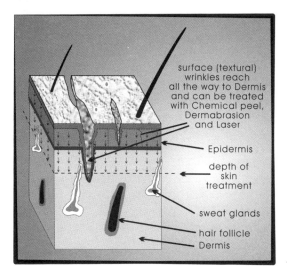

surface (textural) wrinkles reach all the way to Dermis and can be treated with Chemical peel, Dermabrasion and Laser

Epidermis

depth of skin treatment

sweat glands

hair follicle

Dermis

The skin is two layers, the epidermis and the dermis. Hair and sweat glands are lined by epidermis cells, and extend well into the dermis.

4a)

Dermabrasion, chemical peels and laser resurfacing remove the epidermis and part of the dermis, leaving sweat glands and hair follicles in the remaining dermis.

4b)

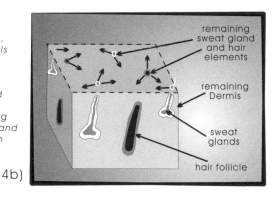

remaining sweat gland and hair elements

remaining Dermis

sweat glands

hair follicle

4c)

wrinkle shallower

new Epidermis thinner

sweat glands

hair follicle

Dermis

Cells grow out from the hair and sweat glands to form a new epidermis. The dermis is slightly thinner. After healing, shallow wrinkles may be eliminated, deeper ones are shallower.

common with cigarete smoking. Many women in their seventies and eighties have smooth skin but exhibit architectural changes of aging such as jowls and neck bands; in contrast, patients who have spent a great deal of time in the sun often have thickened, leathery skin, cross hatched with deep and fine creases and lines. Smokers often have extensive fine line wrinkles running from the mouth outwards and around the eyes.

The skin is made up of two main layers, the epidermis and the dermis. The epidermis is a thin layer which acts as a barrier to prevent moisture from leaving the body and fluid and chemicals from entering the body. The epidermis is several skin cells thick, and which develop from the deepest epidermis, gradually maturing, migrating towards the surface, becoming a keratin protein factory, and finally flaking off at the surface.

Most of the cells in the epidermis are typical skin cells called keratinocytes and their chief function is making keratin, the structural protein of the skin (Many shampoos claim to be enriched with keratin protein, but the value of this is questionable). There are other cells in the epidermis, and these include melanocytes. These make the pigment which gives the skin its colour, and become more active when exposed to the sun, giving a tan. When there has been sun damage, there may be areas of excess pigmentation. Worse, melanocytes are the cells which are linked to melanoma, by far the most serious type of skin cancer, and it is solar radiation which is most responsible for the development of this type of cancer.

The epidermis covers, and is strongly attached to, a much thicker layer, called the dermis. The dermis is a layer of connective tissue with strength and elasticity from two main structural proteins, collagen and elastin and a rich network of blood vessels and lymph channels. Between the dermis and epidermis is a barrier layer called the basement membrane, which is what prevents most commercial anti-wrinkle and anti-cellulite remedies from penetrating to a level where they might have significant effects.

Hair follicles and sweat glands begin in the dermis and end on the surface. They are made up of epidermal cells which extend down into the dermis. This is important in our techniques of skin resurfacing because, with healing, the epidermis must cover the surface, and all resurfacing techniques involve removing the surface of epidermis plus a variable depth of the underlying dermis. The new surface epidermis has to grow out from the hair follicles and sweat glands, and spread out completely to cover the surface once again.

Wrinkles and folds in the skin are really of two types. I try to explain these to patients as deep, architectural changes, requiring surgical repositioning and tightenings for rejuvenation, and surface, or textural changes, which are primarily in the dermis. The surface changes, combined with the thickening and pigmentation changes in the epidermis, are what can be treated with surface procedures.

TREATMENT

Aging and sun damage have been treated for decades with dermabrasion, which is mechanical sanding of the skin with a rapidly spinning abrasive device; or by chemical peel, the application of weak acid solutions. Both methods produce a superficial second degree, or partial thickness burn. Dermabrasion causes a mild friction burn, just as we all got when we fell and scraped ourselves as children; whereas chemical peels produce a mild chemical burn. The original chemical peels in North America were done using Phenol by European estheticians in Miami and were discovered by the medical community in the early 1960's.

Superficial, or Partial thickness burns heal without scarring as long as no infection causes the injury to deepen to deep partial, or full thickness burns. This is true of the scrapes we got as children, of heat induced (thermal) burns, or of chemical burns. The dermis is thinned by the amount which is destroyed by the injury, but the epidermis regenerates from the hair follicles and sweat glands. Initially, the freshly healed epidermis is thin, red, and easily damaged, but it rapidly thickens, gains strength as its attachment to the underlying dermis becomes normal and changes colour to become paler and, if the injury was superficial enough, normally pigmented.

Recently, less aggressive skin treatments including Vitamin A acid and fruit acid (alpha hydroxy acid, or AHA) peels have come into fashion. Dermatologists and estheticians may advocate the use of these agents in regular or even daily skin care routines. Each of these agents may be useful in improving the youthfullness of the skin and reducing the degeneration of skin which may lead to skin cancer. All are somewhat unpredictable and imprecise.

A laser is a device which, simply put, concentrates energy and sends it in a very controlled beam, in such a way that the beam does not spread, and the energy remains concentrated for a considerable distance. If you shine a flashlight, the beam gradually spreads out and the beam of light loses its strength. A laser beam can travel a great distance without scattering or spreading significantly.

Lasers have been used in medicine and surgery for years. However, technology has recently been developed to allow the precise use of lasers for dermatologic and plastic surgical skin rejuvenation. A carbon dioxide laser beam normally vaporizes anything containing water, and thus rapidly cuts through skin and any other organs and structures. Its usefulness as a cutting tool, however, seems to be limited: the bulk and cost of the laser do not seem to be justified by its ability to reduce bleeding and post-operative bruising and pain. Several years ago, after a careful evaluation of the CO_2 laser as a surgical scalpel for cosmetic eye surgery, a noted authority on lasers in plastic surgery concluded the main value of the device was as a promotional tool for the surgeon.

The major innovation of the past few years has been the introduction of pulsing technology, the ability to send very short (less than one thousandth of a second) bursts of CO_2 laser energy to the skin. This will vaporize somewhere between twenty and seventy thousandths of a millimeter of the skin without creating much heat in the deeper tissues, and allows a much more controlled removal of the skin than dermabrasion and chemical peels. There seems to be an additional benefit, which is that the underlying dermis collagen seems to tighten and shrink by about a third, to form a firm, youthful foundation for the new complexion.

The latest development in laser resurfacing is the Erbium:YAG laser, which seems to offer many of the benefits of CO_2 lasers with much faster recovery and less risk of scarring. However, it is too early to know the final results of this laser.

For many plastic surgeons, because of the precision, the bloodless character of the surgery, and the reduced risk of complications, laser resurfacing has replaced chemical peel and dermabrasion.

WHO WOULD BENEFIT FROM LASER SKIN RESURFACING?

Aging skin shows a mixture of dryness, wrinkling, variation in pigmentation, thinning as well as loss of elasticity and sagging. These changes are most dramatic at the surface of sun-damaged skin, and removal of the outer layer, combined with stimulation of new collagen, elastic fibres and development of new epidermis may give profound results. It may be useful alone, or in combination with other esthetic surgery, such as a facelift, forehead lift, or eyelid plasty.

Many facelift patients will benefit from resurfacing around the mouth to reduce the vertical lipstick or smoker lines. The typical shiny, pale result from dermabrasion or peels in this area is rarely seen.

Lower eyelid resurfacing is commonly done with a lower eyelid blepharoplasty done through an incision on the inside of the lid, instead of the traditional approach through an incision under the eyelashes, and the skin tightening done this way seems to have a much lower risk of complications. (see Facial Rejuvenation chapter)

Full face laser resurfacing is now an accepted and widely used treatment for sun-damaged skin, acne scarring, and multiple fine line wrinkles.

RISKS

Although bloodless, laser resurfacing is still a surgical technique. As with any surgery, there are risks. The risks of hypo (under) and hyper (excess) pigmentation are probably significantly less than with traditional resurfacing techniques, but still exist. Creams are prescribed to help to reduce these risks. Infection can occur, and since skin infections most commonly result from bacteria residing in the skin, antibiotics are routinely used for several days after surgery. Viral infection from the cold sore virus (Herpes simplex) can also be re-activated, and because many of us have the virus even if we do not get cold sores, an anti-viral medication is also used routinely, beginning two days prior to the procedure and continuing for several days afterwards. If a cold sore does appear prior to the surgery, the surgery date should be postponed.

Scarring can occur if the depth of the skin removal is excessive, or if infection occurs. Some patients are more at risk for scar and pigmentary problems than others. Generally, fair-skinned individuals have less pigment irregularity than those with darker skin; and patients of Mediterranean heritage are more of a concern than those with Northern European origins, while those with Sino-Asian and black African origins may have too severe a risk of thick scar formation or even keloids (a scar which continues to grow in a tumor like fashion (see Skin Care and Scars chapter) to allow for this treatment. A small "test patch" in an inconspicuous area may determine how you respond if you are at risk for keloid formation.

Although serious complications are unusual, a problem

after laser resurfacing is the redness which occurs in all cases. We expect it to be present for several weeks to three months after the surgery, but on occasion it may last longer - six months or even more. While this can usually be covered with make-up this is a nuisance to patients who lead active lives. It is the main reason why many surgeons advocate full facial resurfacing for most patients, because there is at least a uniform, mildly sunburnt appearance, whereas if only limited areas are done they are more difficult to blend with the surrounding untreated areas. Camouflage cosmetics can be very useful, and the kit I provide to my patients contains a "red-away" preparation.

On rare occasions, patients will experience sensitivity to their usual make-up products early after the healing period. If this occurs, the products should be avoided until further healing takes place, or a substitute should be found.

PREPARATION

As experience has been gained with laser resurfacing, we have realized that results are better and more predictable if the skin is properly prepared. Some believe Vitamin A should be used, others do not. Most routinely believe a product for prevention of excess pigmentation should be used for about two weeks prior to surgery such as hydroquinone or Kojic acid. Careful use of sun blockers is also begun.

THE OPERATION

If laser resurfacing alone is being done, the extent of the procedure may determine the anesthetic technique. For limited areas, application of topical anesthetic cream may be enough, but in most cases it is necessary to inject the anaesthetic solution. As this is uncomfortable, I prefer to have the patients in the operating room properly monitored and lightly sedated with some intra-venous valium-like medications or at least some medications taken by mouth. When a full face treatment is done, especially for acne scarring, where the anaesthetic fluid may not spread well and may miss some areas, deeper sedation or even a general anaesthetic may be more comfortable for the patient. The actual procedure may vary in length from a few minutes to an hour or more, and at the end, a dressing is applied by some surgeons, or the areas may be treated "open" with the application of vaseline or antibiotic ointments.

HEALING

I provide my patients with a kit of skin care products which helps equip them for the post-operative period. We suggest they wash their faces gently and apply an ointment to the treated areas several times a day. They are told to sleep on their backs, and avoid rubbing, scratching or traumatizing the healing areas in any way.

Swelling may be quite significant for the first twenty-four to forty-eight hours, then resolves quite quickly. Increasing pain and swelling after three days may mean that infection has occurred. High fever should also not occur.

A crust initially forms, and healing occurs under the crust, usually in about a week, but some areas may take two weeks. Once the crust comes off it will leave the freshly healed, pink new skin. The next phase of healing takes six to twelve weeks, during which new collagen is made. This helps eliminate the deeper wrinkling and it may be several months before the full effect is seen.

Darker skinned patients may have a period of excess (hyper-) pigmentation and will be treated preventively with hydroquinone and/or Kojic acid.

AFTER HEALING

Normal activity can be resumed as soon as the skin is healed, but it is absolutely vital that the skin be protected from the sun for at least the first year with a good sun block. Of course, in today's environment, this should be a routine for everyone, but special vigilance is needed after resurfacing.

RESHAPING THE FACE

RHINOPLASTY: COSMETIC NOSE SURGERY

Surgery to alter the appearance of the nose has been at the centre of plastic surgery since its earliest days. The history of plastic surgery is intimately related to reconstruction of the nose and discussions of plastic surgery usually mention Tycho Brahe, in the early Renaissance, and his fabricated prosthetic nose; reconstruction of the nose as done in India using the forehead; and the use of the skin of the arm by Tagliacozzi in the 14th century.

Cosmetic surgery, which became a significant field in the 20th century, also has nasal surgery at its roots, with the basics of cosmetic rhinoplasty started by Jacques Joseph in Germany in the 1920's.

The operation has given many patients great satisfaction and increased self esteem but it is regarded by experienced surgeons as one of the most difficult, if not the most difficult, operation in all of surgery. In no other surgery is function (the flow of air through the nasal passages) and form so closely inter-dependent. Furthermore, the nose is always prominent in the middle of the patient's face. In a continuous search for more long-lasting, dependable and predictable results, plastic surgeons are constantly re-evaluating known techniques and working with new ones.

Unfortunately, results are somewhat difficult to evaluate. It takes many months or longer for the consequences of surgery to become clear, and what may look good two or three weeks after surgery may not last over time. Dramatic

57

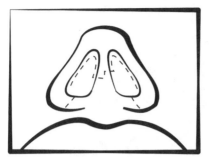

5a)

Rhinoplasty is done through incisions inside the nose, often joined between the nostrils. Incisions may also be needed at the nostril base.

5b)

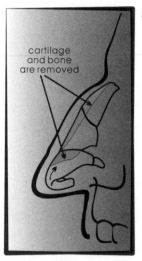

cartilage and bone are removed

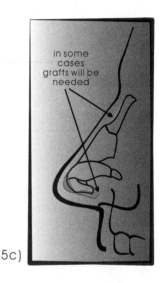

in some cases grafts will be needed

5c)

The bridge may be reduced by removing bone and cartilage. The tip cartilage may be modified to re-shape the tip.

Sometimes grafts of cartilage or bone will be neede to give satisfactory shape and structure.

appearing early results may become unnaturally over-done when final settling occurs months or even years later. However, in the fifty or sixty years in which rhinoplasty for esthetics has been practised, definite trends have developed in surgical philosophy.

Although most patients who request rhinoplasty are concerned with the shape of their nose and usually feel one area or the whole nose is too large, the nose must be

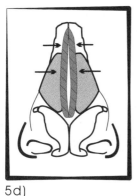 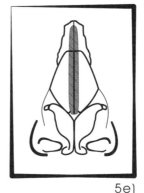

5d) 5e)

The nose may be narrowed by moving the bone and cartilage.

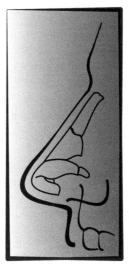

5f)

The resulting nose has more pleasing bridge, tip and angle.

viewed as a complex structure made up of many three dimensional structures which need to blend together with the rest of the face in a harmonious whole. No one operation is right for every patient. The surgery must be carefully planned to respect the need for balance and proportion in each patient. Because of this, the rhinoplasties which were done in earlier years and which are still done by some surgeons which routinely involve reduction of cartilage, shaving off and narrowing the bones, and shortening the nose, will often produce a nose that eventually looks like it has been partially amputated and may even look muti-lated.

In contrast, patients of non-European heritage often have noses which feature small, or thin cartilages and thick skin leading to a nose which is fleshy appearing and lacks definition; one in which the tip is felt to be overly large compared to the bridge. In these noses, the main attention is directed toward augmenting the bridge and middle third, while giving the tip a narrower, better defined shape. This is often accomplished using an implant of man-made materials, although in some cases it may be done with cartilage or bone grafts.

The modern approach has gradually been developed through the experience and teaching of surgeons such as Jack Sheen (in Los Angeles) and George Peck (in New Jersey) beginning in the 1970's, and, later, with a group of surgeons in Dallas (particularly Jack Gunter). This involves selective, subtle reduction and refinement of the bone and cartilage combined, where appropriate, with selective augmentation with cartilage grafts. The key to this concept is that no two noses are alike, and therefore, each nose must be assessed carefully as the sum of many parts, and a part of the face. The aim is to create a nose which has balanced and harmonious components and is itself in balance and harmony with the rest of the face.

This does not necessarily mean reducing the size of a nose which looks too large. This appearance may be an optical illusion created, for example, by a nasal bridge which is disproportionately low and wide for the tip region. Instead of reducing the tip which may result in an operated upon look, the surgeon may feel augmenting the bridge area may restore balance and maintain a natural appearance. I have often used Meryl Streep's nose as an example of one which has grace and proportion giving an appearance of beauty without being small.

For a surgeon, deciding whether or not to operate, is probably more difficult in rhinoplasty surgery than in almost any other area of esthetic surgery, for several reasons. The psychological effects of a nose which is seen to be unsightly by the patient have likely been present for many years, often since early adolescence. Among other factors, the patient may have been teased by peers, or felt rejected emotionally, or felt to be ethnically conspicuous. Expectations of the operation may run unrealistically high, and because the effects of surgery do not appear immediately, disappointment may set in and be persistent.

The surgeon must try to select the patients who can understand the aims of surgery in their individual case, along with the limits to what can be performed. A host of factors determine the outcome of surgery, only some of which are under the control of the surgeon. These include the texture and thickness of the skin, the strength and size of the underlying bone and cartilage and the age of the patient, among others. But it is not just the combination of factors involved, and the shape of the patient's nose prior to surgery which determine the final outcome. The patient's concern may be the most important factor, and this is often not easy to determine in pre-operative discussions. Concern with small details may be either the warning of a patient who will never be satisfied, or may indicate one who will appreciate a good result. Obsession with detail, on the contrary, indicates the patient will likely not be satisfied, given that small imperfections result from nearly every operation. If definite, relatively predictable surgical maneuvers will likely give the kind of shape the patient desires, and if the patient expresses these desires clearly and without obsessiveness, there is a high chance of success.

The functional aspects of the nose must also be considered. The flow of air through the nose may be unsatisfactory prior to surgery due to development or to previous injuries such as a broken nose. There may be reduced airflow due to allergies and chronic inflammation, and these will not be helped by surgery. In cocaine users, the wall running down the centre of the inside of the nose (the septum) may develop a hole, or perforation, and at an extreme, the nose may collapse due to loss of support from the septum. There are other illnesses which may cause problems with the function of the nose, and these need to be discussed with your doctor, diagnosed, and treated, if possible.

Surgery may, in part, aim to improve the flow of air but in reducing the size of the nose the flow of air may be reduced and some measures may have to be taken to improve this. The nose may appear nearly straight, but a twist or bend in the septum, may become more apparent as the bridge of the nose is reduced. Making a crooked nose perfectly straight is exceedingly difficult although much can be done to improve the alignment of the nasal architecture. Patients who want their noses reduced beyond what is likely compatible with function and those who want a perfect nose when it is slightly or completely crooked prior to surgery, should likely not undergo surgery.

THE OPERATION

Traditionally, cosmetic nasal surgery was done entirely through incisions inside the nose, with the exception of small ones at the base of the nostrils. Very often local anesthesia, only, was used. Because they performed a stereotyped operation, and under local anaesthesia, surgeons sometimes prided themselves that the operation did not take more than twenty or thirty minutes. Often the incisions were left to heal without stitches. A plaster cast was placed on the nose and often extended up onto the forehead and out onto the cheeks. Gauze bandage, or packing, one half to one inch wide and a foot or longer in length, was nearly always placed in the nose, and left for two days to up to a week, and patients were usually kept in hospital at least for the first night after surgery.

Today, depending on the patient, the operation is done either under local or general anaesthesia but it is nearly always done on an outpatient basis. Many surgeons have added a small incision between the nostrils to the inside incisions, giving greater control over the way the tip can be shaped, because the complex shape of the tip cartilages can be better assessed and changed accurately under direct vision. Structures higher up in the nose can also be seen better than they could through the traditional key-hole incisions inside the nose. External splints are smaller, thinner and lighter, and internal thin plastic splints or stitching replaces packing in many cases, or at least limits its use to a very short period.

The external splint is usually removed at five to seven days at which time the external stitches are also removed. At this time there is usually still some crusting and fullness in the nostrils which gradually clears. This may be aided by frequent application of antibiotic ointment to reduce drying and crusting. Sneezing through the nose should be avoided if possible.

I generally tell patients they can expect to be back to work in seven to ten days, by which time most of the bruising has resolved. Light exercise can start at two weeks and full sports at six. Although it is an approximation, I tell them swelling takes at least six months to finally resolve, although it is about sixty percent gone at two weeks, and ninety per cent at six weeks.

COMPLICATIONS

As with any surgery, bleeding, infection and changes of sensation are potential problems. Infection is highly unusual, and bleeding requiring treatment occurs in about one per cent of cases, although it is normal to have slight post-operative bleeding for the first day or so after surgery. It is highly unusual to have any significant alteration in the sense of smell subsequent to surgery. Sensation of the tip of the nose is usually temporarily reduced and the nose will feel stiff and rather numb for several months after the surgery. Some cold sensitivity during the first winter after surgery is common.

The flow of air through the nose may be altered by surgery. Any surgery to the nose can alter the flow of air, although we generally aim to improve the flow- but any attempt to narrow the nose, especially, can reduce the flow. In fact, reduced flow can result from any of a variety of factors. The sensation of reduced flow can even, strangely enough, result from improving the flow of air, on occasion, because a patient who is used to feeling the turbulence of reduced airflow through the nose may not feel anything when breathing is without obstruction, and may be under the illusion there is no flow.

The most common problem from rhinoplasty surgery is dissatisfaction with the esthetic result. In many cases this can be remedied with secondary surgery, and when the source of dissatisfaction is well-defined, and there is a clear anatomic solution, ultimate satisfaction is usually the result of secondary surgery. However, when the cartilages and other structures have been reduced and are deficient, reconstruction may be a difficult matter. All plastic surgeons see patients from time to time who have had previous rhinoplastic surgery and are dissatisfied. In most cases, it is helpful to have the old operative reports. Sometimes the surgeon who performed the original surgery is best able to do the secondary procedure, partially because he or she knows what was done previously, and knows what is available for secondary surgery. In general, because the final shape from a rhinoplasty is not achieved until all swelling has resolved and scar healing is complete, it is best not to contemplate revision until at least six months have passed since the original procedure.

I have seen numerous patients who expressed some initial dissatisfaction with the result at four to six weeks after surgery and were reassured that there was still significant swelling; by six months after surgery many of their concerns had resolved. As with many other plastic surgical procedures, patience is rewarded.

OTOPLASTY: SURGERY OF OUTSTANDING EARS

Probably no younger patients come to the attention of the surgeon performing cosmetic facial surgery than those with prominent ears. Because prominent ears are noticed early in childhood and quickly become the objects of ridicule from other children, it is most common for parents to bring children to a consultation soon after a child begins pre-school, and most surgery to set back the ears is done in childhood.

Because the ridicule and abuse directed at a child with outstanding ears is significant, medical insurance will generally cover the cost of surgery on children, which generally means up the age of sixteen.

The satisfaction rate with this type of surgery is very high, and the rate of major complications is very low. Even when a patient has come through childhood without having undergone surgery, and finally decides to opt for surgery, it is unusual to have significant dissatisfaction with the surgery, and most patients are thrilled with the results.

The typical patient comes with a story that he or she has never felt comfortable with shorter hair styles, and is very self conscious about his or her appearance.

Historically, there have been many operations devised to make the ears less prominent, and there continue to be many different ways to achieve reasonably similar anatomical goals.

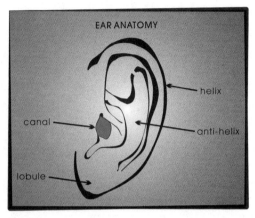

6a)
Ear anatomy

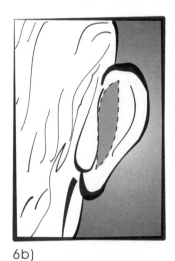

6b)

An incision is made behind the ear to give access to the ear cartilage.

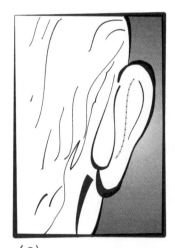

6c)

Reshaping of the ear cartilages gives it a more pleasing angle and size.

ANATOMY

Although many patients come complaining that their ears are too large, it is highly unusual for the actual vertical and horizontal dimensions to be outside the range of normal. The ear ranges from about 5.5 to 7.5 centimeters in length. It is unusual even in patients who have "big ears", for these measurements to be exceeded. What a plastic surgeon sees is different. The distance of the outer edge of the ear to the side of the head is where the ear becomes different in patients who want their ears set back. Patients generally start to see the ears as being out of proportion when this distance becomes greater than about two centimeters.

The outer ear, which is what concerns the patient, is made up of skin covering a very complex cartilage shape, with many prominences and hollows:

> The helix, which is the rolled rim.
> The antihelix, a convex roll in the middle of the ear, branching in two towards the top.
> The scapha, a long hollow between the helix and anti-helix.
> The concha (from the greek, seashell), the bowl - like depression in the middle.
> The tragus, a little bump in front of the ear canal.
> The Ear canal, the tunnel leading to the middle and inner ear.
> The lobule, the fleshy portion at the bottom from which earrings hang.

As we see in the diagram, the ear cartilage folds determine how far the ear protrudes from the side of the head. A fold at the anti-helix bends the ear back toward the side of the head; when this fold is very slight or absent, the ear curls away from the head sticks out more than usual.

There may also be a deeper concha, the bowl-shaped area immediately next to the ear canal, and this may cause the ear to protrude.

TREATMENT

Otoplasty may be performed on an out-patient basis in a private operating room setting. It rarely requires an overnight stay. The surgery takes one to two hours, and may be done under general or twilight anesthesia combined with local.

There are many surgical techniques for setting the ears back into a normal distance from the side of the head. Most involve creating a greater curve to the anti-helix and may involve reducing the depth of the concha. Some other, smaller alterations to the cartilage may also be involved.

Usually the operation involves removing some skin from the back of the ear, which, when the ear is folded back, will be excessive. The main efforts are directed towards re-shaping the cartilage. To do this the surgeon usually first makes it more flexible. This may be done by cutting, scoring, or rasping (which is like filing with a rough instument). This alone may cause the cartilage to curl, but often stitches are used to give a controlled curve and these may be permanent or semi-permanent stitches under the back surface, or may be external stiches used to hold the shape for ten to fourteen days. If the concha is deep, a small crescent of cartilage may be removed, again from the back of the ear, and the cut cartilage edges are stitched. The incision behind the ear is closed, and a bulky head bandage is applied. After a brief period in the recovery room, the patient is usually discharged.

POST-OPERATIVE CARE

The major risks of surgery are similar to the risks of any other surgery, including bleeding, infection, nerve injury, and loss of feeling. All of these are rare. Severe pain not responding to the usual pain killers in the first twenty-four to forty-eight hours may indicate pressure build-up from bleeding; gradually or suddenly worsening pain after the first day may mean infection.

Many patients ask me if the surgery will affect their hearing. Because the outer ear is not the hearing organ, which is deep in the head at the end of the ear canal, the short answer to this question is no. But if you cup your ear with your hand while listening you will hear a change, and making the ear less outstanding from the side of the head will have a small effect on the quality of sound.

I usually see otoplasty patients the first or second day after surgery and change the dressing. A fresh, soft bandage is more comfortable, and is left on for the remainder of a week, after which the stitches behind the ear are removed.

I suggest to patients that once the dressing is removed they wear an athletic headband over the ears at night for about three weeks, to prevent deforming the ear when sleeping. Much of the swelling goes down quickly, so the ears look near normal within a week to ten days, but the final shape is not seen for months.

LIP AUGMENTATION AND REDUCTION

The mouth, brow, and eyes are responsible for forming most of the facial expressions by which we communicate our emotions. Traditionally, thin lips were said to be a sign of anger, a lacking of compassion, and of cold emotion. Pursing the lips is a sign of disapproval. Bearing these concepts in mind, the current interest in lip augmentation is likely based on two factors.

The first is the obvious inter-racial concepts of beauty being promoted in the fashion press especially seen in the strong photo-fashion journalism of such magazines as ELLE, which from its inception in the mid-1980's gave models, who obviously had mixed and non-European racial heritage, strong representation. This has obviously reflected and made more universal a concept of beauty which does not necessarily reflect the classic canons. In no area is this as obvious as in the fullness of the models' lips. At first this was exclusively due to inherited characteristics. Unfortunately, it is now obvious how many models have been surgically augmented to extremes. The presumed esthetic reason for having augmented lips in young women is that full lips are sensuous-appearing, and, perhaps, international / inter-racial.

The second factor, once again, is the increased understanding of what elements contribute to the appearance of youth, and the importance of the smile and the area around the mouth to the impression of youth. When we see

7a)

Lip Anatomy: The vermillion is the red area of lips where lipstick is normally applied.

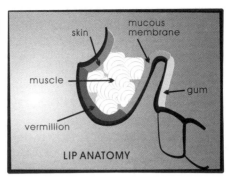

LIP ANATOMY

7b)

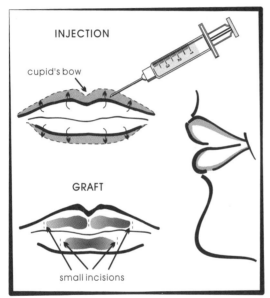

The volume of the lips may be increased by injection or by the placement of grafts. The vermillion (red portion) may be brought outward (arrows) to increase the amount of vermillion showing.

7c)

V-to-Y advancements can be done from the inside to increase the amount of vermillion showing.

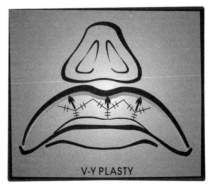

V-Y PLASTY

a person whose face looks old, among the areas which give that impression are the loss of youthful teeth, the appearance of vertical lines running from the lip outwards, thinning of the lips and reduction of the reddish-pink "vermillion" of the lips.

Augmentation of the lips only became a popular plastic surgical procedure in the late 1980's. I recall getting many telephone calls about lip enhancement shortly after the release of a movie in which one of the female leads had obviously undergone a lip enhancement; it suddenly became obvious to the public that this was an area which was also open to improvement by cosmetic surgery.

Since that time I have seen many forms of lip augmentation suggested and practised by members of the cosmetic surgical community, but most of the procedures are not be acceptable to me for a variety of reasons.

In order to discuss lip augmentation, I usually find it necessary to describe the anatomy in fair detail so that the aims and limitations of surgery are clear.

The surfaces of the lip are covered with skin on the outside, mucous membrane inside, and the vermillion, a transition type of skin, between. Generally, most patients desire more vermillion to show as a band of red across the lip, and this can be achieved, to some extent, by applying lipstick beyond the border between the skin and the vermillion (the vermillion margin) or even by tattooing this area; they also want fuller, thicker lips, and this means the distance from the mucous membrane lining the lip and skin on the outside is greater. Many also want the shape of the cupid's bow, the gently undulating upper lip border with the skin, to be accentuated. If there are fine lines radiating outward from the lips, this may cause lipstick to "bleed" or run up the lines, obscuring the definition, which is one of the aims of lipstick.

My approach to lip augmentation is first to decide what aspects of these factors are most important to the patient. I then review the various treatment modes which have been, and are, available. I usually divide these into three broad categories:

1. Injections
   liquid silicone (banned)
   collagen proteins
   microsphere plastic suspensions
   *Fat taken from the patient

2. Implants
   Gore-tex (W.L. Gore & assoc., Flagstaff Arizona) strips
   Cadaver dermis (available commercially)
   *Fascia (a tough, flexible material which can be taken from the surface of the patient's own muscle through small incisions
   *Dermis-, or dermis-fat grafts (taken from the patient)

3. Incisions
   "Lip Roll" procedure
   *"V-Y plasty" procedure

*My preferred methods

The most popular of these procedures over the years among surgeons and dermatologists have been the injection of silicone, collagen, and fat, and the lip roll and V-Y plasty procedures.

A few words, and just a few, about the use of collagen. I gave up on collagen nearly five years ago for both lips and wrinkles. I found that in order to give my patients the kind of lip increase they wanted, it required the use of several syringe-fulls of collagen at several hundred dollars per syringe. Furthermore, the collagen seemed to disappear from the lip much more quickly than from other locations. Instead of lasting three to six months, which is about how long it plumps the skin when used for wrinkles, it seemed to disappear in four to six weeks at the most. There have also been scattered reports about significant health effects from the use of collagen and my feeling has been that the benefits of collagen are limited. The cost to the patient is high, so even a small risk seems difficult for me to justify.

I have not seen Gore-tex augmented lips which felt natural and my patients who have had it implanted by other surgeons generally are less than pleased with the result. Most patients from the Pacific Northwest are not interested in using Gore-tex for anything other than shedding the ever-present rain, a use for which it excels.

Finally, the lip roll procedure, which involves removing a complete or nearly complete thin strip of skin from above the vermillion margin, and pulling the vermillion up to fill the resulting space. This sounds good in theory but in practice results in a scar which takes a long time to fade and doesn't really address the fundamental concern of the patient.

Most patients want a fuller look, if possible with the presence of a pout a la Brigitte Bardot. Hence, the term "Paris Lip", coined by the manufacturers of collagen. Increased vermillion show is also desired but seems to be a secondary goal.

To give a fuller lip, I feel the need to address the volume of the lip directly. In other words, something needs to be added, because the lips are either thin, to begin with, or have thinned with age. As the volume of the lip increases, so does the degree to which the vermillion is visible. To add volume, I use a graft, a transplant from elsewhere in the body, because this makes use of the patient's own tissues, and once the graft develops its own nourishing blood supply, it becomes incorporated in the new site. The main problem with this type of procedure is how much graft is going to survive. And taking the graft requires a donor site. Depending on the procedure, this may result in a tiny scar (fat injection) or a fine line scar of two to three inches in a concealed area (dermis-fat grafting). On rare occasions, I have also done a V-Y plasty procedure to increase vermillion show after increasing the lip volume; I have also occasionally used grafts from material removed during a facelift, or fascia from the temple, in a manner similar to that used in dermis-fat grafting. However, by far the most common methods used are fat grafting and dermis-fat grafts.

In fat injections, an area of the abdomen, buttocks or thigh is anesthetised with local anesthetic, and a little liposuction is done to harvest the fat. The fat is then washed with saline and filtered through a screen to remove broken fat cells and blood. The fat is loaded into a syringe, and injected into the lips which have also been anesthetized. The entire procedure takes only about half an hour. Pain is minimal and the chance of post-operative problems with infection and bleeding is minimal; I have never seen either. I warn the patients that they walk out of the clinic looking like Daisy Duck, because it is necessary to put in a large volume of fat, of which only ten to twenty percent survives. The excess gradually goes down over the ensuing week, and final results are seen at six to eight weeks. How much of the fat survives varies from patient to patient. Usually about 15% to 25% survival can be expected. The procedure can be repeated until a desirable increase is achieved.

With the dermis-fat procedure, the aim is to achieve a lasting result in one or two sessions. Here, the graft, taken from a concealed area, consists of a strip of skin from which the thin surface layer (the epi-dermis) has been removed, and the underlying dermis with its attached fat, is pre-shaped, and then inserted through tiny incisions, into tunnels formed in the lips. In this procedure, I expect thirty to fifty percent survival of the graft, so again, I over compensate and there is initial excess fullness. In the absence of infection, the graft generally shrinks uniformly, so when I say thirty to fifty percent survival, this does not mean one hundred percent on one side and zero on the other. The major drawback of this operation is the donor site scar, and techniques are being developed for harvesting strips of dermis from under the epidermis with a coring device, so as not to leave a surface scar. There is also a slightly higher risk of infection in comparison with the fat injection procedure.

This operation is also usually done under local anesthesia,

and takes me about one hour to perform. Patients are generally given some sedation but this is not necessary.

The final procedure, V-Y plasty, which is done frequently by some other surgeons, is one which I reserve for special circumstances where the vermillion show is still not sufficient after either or both of the above. Most of the patients I have seen who have had this done say there is a prolonged period during which their lips felt stiff and unnatural during which the scars, which are inside of the lip, are healing and maturing. This operation makes use of a classic plastic surgical technique for shifting tissue.

When a V-shaped incision is made and then stitched up to form a Y, the central area is pushed away from the lower leg of the Y. If several V's linked in a zig-zag pattern on the inside of the lip, and then closed in a series of connected Y's with the central areas towards the vermillion and the lower legs of the Y's towards the inside, the result is that the vermillion is pushed outwards. In principle and in practice, this works very well, but as I have explained, it is best also to increase the lip bulk first. However, the discomfort and temporary unnatural feeling resulting from the surgery makes this a secondary choice of procedure to me.

ADDITIONAL CONSIDERATIONS

The position and shape of the lips is determined, to a large extent, by the shape of the underlying teeth and jaws. Patients who have a narrow arch of teeth, a small upper jaw, and those who have had teeth removed or pushed back, will have lips that appear less full. Where the patient has been wearing dentures for many years, the bone which surrounded the teeth will have disappeared, and no surgical procedure on the lips alone will restore youthful fullness. In some cases, a complete dental restoration programme should be considered, especially now that the success of dental implants has been established.

The fine line wrinkles around the mouth will not disappear

with either a lip augmentation or a facelift. The texture and quality of the skin has been lost, and the lines can only be reduced by working directly on the skin along with with the lip augmentation. This is done by means of a re-surfacing procedure, chemical or laser peel which results in healing with a smoother surface.

LIP REDUCTION

Lips can be made less prominent by reducing the soft tissues of the lips, including mucous membrane (lining), vermillion, and the deep tissues of the lips, and can be quite effective, with a low risk of complications. Mucous membranes are particularly good areas for scar formation. The scars settle quite rapidly and keloid formation is rare, even in patients at risk (see Skin Care and Scars chapter).

FACIAL BONE SURGERY

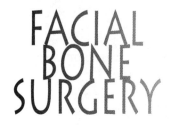

Through the ages, artists have attempted to define perfection in facial appearance but the definition of beauty along strict, measurable terms has always been difficult and may be impossible. The Greeks believed that classical beauty embodied precise but balanced measurements: The harmonious proportion of facial features was often thought the secret to facial beauty. Plato saw the structure of the human body and face as a system of triads and centuries later observers sought the mathematical formula to define beauty. By the Renaissance, however, this ideal had changed. Francis Bacon wrote that "there is no excellent beauty that hath not some strangeness in its proportions."

Although there would seem to be cultural bias as to what constitutes the most attractive proportions between the various facial features, one could argue that faces are most pleasing when they demonstrate a similar harmony of proportions to that seen in nature, especially in the repetitive occurrence of the so-called "golden rectangles" and "divine proportions." Many plastic surgeons have continued in the classic search to define beauty and have used the classical canons of beauty, as described by Albrecht Durer, Leonardo da Vinci and others, to aid in shaping the facial bony features to give an overall appearance of beauty. The argument is made that these proportions have universal appeal, and are seen implicitly in the forms of many beautiful things in nature (such as the spirals of sea shells) and in classically beautiful architecture such as the Parthenon. We respond to these portions in the faces and bodies of individuals we consider to be attractive or beautiful. Balance and harmony provide a sense of completeness and stability, freed from visual tension and distortion. The Greeks believed that all beauty was based on mathematics and that beautiful objects could be analyzed by numbers. For them, a form such as a rectangle with sides of 1:1.6 was aesthetically the most satisfying. Unfortunately, absolute numbers are of uncertain value when trying to determine nose size and shape on a small thin face or large round one. Perhaps Keats was right when he declared "Beauty is truth, truth beauty."

Plastic Surgery has looked to Anthropologists who have measured multiple angles and proportions on many faces from different cultures, in order to create a guide for the plastic surgeon. This "anthropometric" study has some value, but it may be both misleading and somewhat rigid, and plastic surgeons tend to use both the classic canons of beauty and the modern anthropometric studies less as rigid rules than as a general guide.

In general, the facial profile is divided into thirds which are roughly equal, and when one third is obviously out of proportion to the others, a method of improving the balance is suggested. Similarly, in profile, the forehead, lips and chin are ideally felt to align, the underside of the nose and upper lip form an angle of $100°$ to $110°$. When viewed from the front, the eyes are felt to be best separated from their inner corners (the inner canthi) by about the width of one eye, and the total width of the face at the level of the eyes is about four eye widths (each eye, the distance between them, and half that measure beyond each eye to the sides).

In practice, however, patients do come seeking advice about chins which are small or large, cheekbones which are lacking prominence, and overall facial shapes which would be considered unattractive, in any culture. Often, these individuals have endured ridicule from early school age, and seek relief from the prejudices which surround them.

Literature is full of characters who have been mistreated

because of appearance, and even today, some features are wrongly associated with crudeness and low intelligence (such as a severely protruding lower jaw), or weakness of character (such as a receding jaw or chin). The same is true in politics and in the performing arts.

There are many syndromes which are associated with facial deformities which may be found in patients with normal intelligence: some are even associated with learning and mental disabilities. The treatment of facial deformities is a field of reconstructive plastic surgery which has evolved dramatically in the past twenty-five years following the pioneering work of Paul Tessier, who is widely regarded as the father of modern day "Craniofacial surgery." The scope of this surgery is well beyond the aims of this book, except to say that many of the concepts which began in reconstructive surgery have gradually come to be applied to esthetic facial surgery. These include the concept that entire blocks of the facial bones can be moved and secured in a new position without endangering their nutrition and survival; by means of this concept, when necessary, radical changes in the shape of the face can be made.

However, for the most part, plastic surgeons treat more subtle degrees of facial disharmony, and this may be accomplished either by the use of man-made implants to the chin, cheeks, or other, less common areas, or by modifying the existing bony contours.

CHIN AND CHEEK AUGMENTATION

The most commonly done procedures involve camouflaging areas where bones are relatively small by adding an implant which is made of solid silicone rubber, porous polyethylene, or other plastic-like substance. Many patients undergoing nose surgery have a chin implant placed at the same time; a receding chin seems to occur very frequently in association with a hooked nose, and often the balance produced by adding a chin implant allows a lesser and more natural reduction of the nose.

A chin implant may be placed through an incision inside the mouth where it leaves no visible scar, or under the chin, where it is well concealed. After years of using an incision inside the mouth, I now usually use one under the chin because it gives more reliable placement of the implant at the level we desire, and the risk of having the implant positioned asymmetrically is substantially less. I also use an implant with what is called an anatomic design, which wraps well around the jaw and extends down the sides, to blend with the pre-existing jawline. Other designs only add to the chin button itself, and I have removed and replaced many with better designs because of their unnatural appearance.

Cheek implants are made of similar materials and may be selected from several designs, depending on what part of the middle face is felt to benefit from augmentation. Several incision routes are described for the placement of the implants. They may be put in through the same incision and at the same time as a face lift, or lower eyelid blepharoplasty, either through the outside or inside of the eyelid. Most commonly, however, they are placed through incisions inside the mouth. This may be done under local or general anesthesia.

RISKS AND POSSIBLE COMPLICATIONONS

Infection: As with any foreign material, if post-operative infection occurs in the presence of an implant, it may be necessary to remove the implant in order to cure the infection. Often, however, if infection is treated early enough and aggressively enough, the implant may be salvaged.

Numbness: Because the implant is placed in close proximity to the nerves which give feeling to the lower lip and chin, or

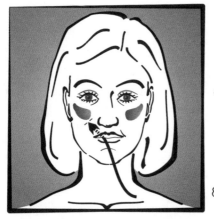

Cheek implants are usually placed through incisions in the mouth, although lower eyelid incisions may be used. They are also sometimes placed during a facelift.

8a)

8b)

8c)

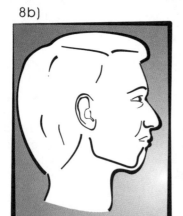

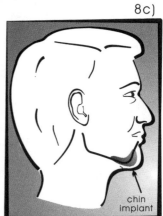

chin implant

A chin implant is usually placed through an incision under the chin, although some surgeons prefer to use an incision in the mouth.

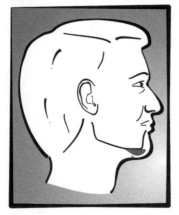

An alternative to chin implants is bone genioplasty. The chin bone is cut horizontally and the lowest portion is slid forward like a drawer.

8d)

upper lip in the case of cheek implants, it is possible to have post-operative numbness, although this is rarely permanent. Significant problems with bleeding are rare, in the absence of an underlying bleeding disorder.

Bony Changes: Because the implant lies in direct contact with the jaw bone, and the overlying muscles exert pressure on it, the implant may cause the underlying bone to absorb and the implant may sink back into the bone a millimeter or even more. If the implant is positioned correctly, over the thick, hard bone of the lower chin, this is not a problem. However, if the implant lies too high it may rest on the thin bone surrounding the tooth roots, and erosion of the bone can occur leading to problems with the teeth. This is not seen with cheek implantation.

Loss of the Implant: Extrusion, the implant becoming exposed at the site of the original incision, or even at another point, may be seen, and requires removal of the implant, This complication, fortunately, is rare.

OTHER PROCEDURES

GENIOPLASTY OR SLIDING OSTEOTOMY OF THE CHIN

Because of the problems seen with implant use, and the limitations as to the amount of augmentation which can be achieved through their use, and also because some patients are adverse to the use of man-made substances in the implants, augmentation of the chin can be achieved through the use of chin bone re-positioning techniques. Essentially, this involves making an incision through the bone horizontally, about one centimeter above the bottom of the chin, and sliding the lower portion of the jaw forward like a drawer. It is then fixed in the new, advanced position by the use of fine bone screws or wires, which hold it until the bone has united. The metal fixation devices rarely require removal.

MAJOR ADVANCEMENT OR SETBACK OF THE JAW OR JAWS

When the jaws have so much inequality that the teeth fail to meet in a functional manner, the upper teeth may be far ahead of the lowers, or vice versa. There are cosmetic and functional results of this. When mild, this may be treated by orthodontics (tooth braces) alone, but sometimes surgery is required to correct adequately a dento-facial deformity. This may involve moving the lower jaw, the upper jaw, or both, depending on the desired esthetic and functional outcome. Usually, it requires somewhere between six and eighteen months of pre-surgical orthodontics, during which time the way the teeth meet together may actually be temporarily made worse in preparation for the bony shift, and six to twelve months of post-surgical treatment to make final fine adjustments to the teeth. This results of this type of surgery may be dramatic, but it is bigger surgery and the risks and possibilities of post-operative problems are greater. Added to the usual risks of bleeding and infection are the higher risks of loss of sensation, failure of the cut edges of bone to heal(requiring bone grafting), and problems with the final meeting and function of the teeth. This type of surgery requires a major commitment on the patient's part, as well as excellent team work between the orthodontist, the surgeon, who may be a plastic surgeon or an oral-maxillo-facial surgeon (dentist specializing in dental surgery), and often other dental specialists such as the prosthedontist, who may help the orthodontist and the surgeon in planning the surgery and completing the post-surgical care.

Bones such as the brow ridge maybe slightly modified to give a rounder, smoother appearance, by removal of some bony prominences.

BONY AUGMENTATION,
BONY EXPANSION

This is an area of continuing intense research in plastic surgery. Bone grafts in the face have been used for many years for reconstructive purposes. A segment of bone is taken from the outer layer of the skull, a rib, or part of the hip and transferred to an area where it is needed, gains a nutritional blood supply and becomes joined to the surrounding bone. Unfortunately, this method often results in loss of substantial amount of bone over time in certain areas where the bone is not needed to do any work. The cheek bone prominences, for example, are notorious for having bone grafts gradually disappear over time. This is felt to be because, unlike a graft to an area like a poorly healing broken leg, the cheek grafts merely sit in position without doing any work (a good example of "use it or lose it").

Research is being done in plastic surgery centres into the concept of gradually changing the shape of bones by cutting them and applying traction with expansion devices, and significant results have already been obtained in lengthening profoundly underdeveloped jaws. (This "Illizarov" method, was pioneered in Russia for leg length problems) Currently, these techniques are just starting to be used for reconstructive surgery of facial deformities. It is quite possible that this will be the way of the future, possibly displacing current jaw surgery techniques, but it will be some time before the techniques will have been refined enough to consider using in esthetic surgical patients.

BREAST AND BODY SURGERY

BREAST AUGMENTATION

Enhancement of the breast by placement of an artificial device, a prosthesis or implant, has been done since the early 1960's by plastic surgeons. Complications are fortunately few, and most are treatable to a satisfactory conclusion. As with any procedure being done very often (and there are likely over two million women who have breast implants) cases of major problems will and do occur.

Despite a storm of controversy which has hovered around the operation since its inception, it continues to satisfy the vast majority of patients. Although the procedure does not always result in excellent results, only a very small proportion of those having the surgery would even consider having the implants removed, and satisfaction rates with both surgeon and patients are high. Despite this, the controversy which has surrounded the operation has forced a re-evaluation and careful assessment of the success of surgery. The long-term results of the surgery are under more careful study than they were previously. Fortunately, the general impression we have always had which is that it is a rewarding procedure, has largely been reinforced by the current studies.

The patient coming for augmentation is usually either in her early twenties, who has very little breast development, often with siblings aunts or mother who have significantly larger breast size; or is in her thirties and has loss of breast volume after having gone through one or several pregnancies and breast feeding periods.

In the 1950's some women, usually involved in burlesque shows or in the US entertainment industry, wanting increase in the size of their breasts, were treated outside North America, by the injection of materials such as liquid silicone or paraffin, directly into the breast, often with rather disastrous results. They experienced painful cyst formation, drainage of infected material, and distortion of the breast shape, so surgeons in North America began searching for reliable and reasonably safe ways of increasing the breast size. This resulted in the develop-

9a

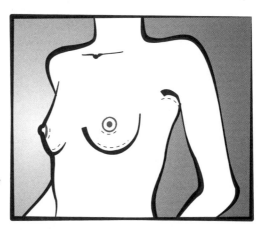

An incision is made in the crease under the breast, at the edge of the areola (the darker skin around the nipple), or in the armpit.

9b)

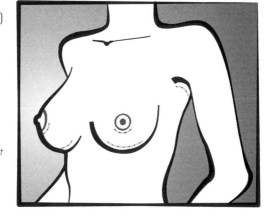

The post-operative result with fuller breasts.

ment of an implant with a silicone rubber shell, or balloon, which could be filled with either silicone gel material manufactured to have approximately the same feel as normal breast tissue, filled at the time of surgery with sterile salt water (saline) or another liquid material no longer used (dextran solution). Instead of entering the breast gland itself, the implant was placed under the breast, leaving the breast, nipple, and areola, essentially intact.

The operation was gradually refined and some modifications were introduced, but it is essentially the same in principle today. While gel-filled implants are no longer available (more about that later), the silicone rubber shell remains, as does the principle of placing the implant under the breast. To understand the dimensional changes, we can think of the operation as one which essentially takes a roughly cone-shaped part of the body (the breast) and increases both the base and its forward projection by adding a round disc (the implant) to the base of the cone.

RISK & POSSIBLE COMPLICATIONS

As with any surgical procedure, breast augmentation can result in bleeding, which though unusual, does occur occasionally. Because a rather large space is created under the breast to allow placement of the implant, if post-operative bleeding occurs under the surface, it can accumulate to a significant amount and cause painful swelling and require urgent treatment. This usually involves a return to the operating room which may mean admission to hospital.

Although infection is highly unusual, it can occur, and if it does, may require removal of the implant for a period of several months until everything is completely settled, followed by re-augmentation.

Loss of feeling or reduced feeling of the breast and nipple occurs more frequently, probably in 15% or more of patients. Although feeling usually gradually returns, it may not, or it may result in increased sensitivity for several months.

CAPSULAR CONTRACTURE

With experience, surgeons recognized that there is one problem which continues to be the main challenge.

Whenever a foreign material, whether it is a sliver, a piece of glass, shrapnel, or a breast implant is placed under the surface of the body, the body recognizes it as not part of itself, and if it cannot digest it, reacts by forming a wall around it. This wall, which we call a capsule, is very much like scar, and may be thin and soft, or tough and thick. In the early phases of healing, all scars contract. If the capsule contracts around the implant and the space available to the implant becomes tight, the implant comes under pressure, is forced into a more rounded shape, and becomes firm or even hard. This condition, which we call capsular contracture, is by far the most common problem for both plastic surgeons doing breast augmentation and our patients. We cannot explain why one patient will get contractures and another will not, nor why in some patients one side will develop a contracture and the other will not. Nor can we predict who will get the condition.It poses no major health risk to the patient but may cause enough firmness on occasion to be uncomfortable or even painful and certainly, the more severe, the less natural they appear and feel.

We generally find that 75-80% of patients have a very good to excellent result, and of the other 20-25%, most have an acceptably soft breast result. A smaller number, perhaps 5-10% may require a secondary operation to help improve the result and a very small number have persistent problems despite all efforts, yet incredibly few patients are troubled enough to want to have their implants removed for treatment of contracture.

Many solutions have been tried with few successes. In earlier days of breast augmentation, surgeons used cortisone and similar medications in and around the implant to reduce scar formation, but this resulted in unreasonable numbers of patients having implants break through the skin or the surgical incision site, requiring removal. Antibiotics were placed in and around the implant on the theory that unrecognized low grade infection, or at least contamination with normal skin bacteria, caused the contractures. However, this brought little or no success. Many surgeons, and their patients believe that contracture can be warded off by daily exercises to keep the implant moving within a space larger than the implant, to maintain a large, relaxed space. In the early 1980's, some surgeons came to believe strongly that placing the implant beneath the breast and the underlying pectoral muscle resulted in a reliably smaller chance of contracture. Because the muscles are being used constantly, so the theory goes, the implant is constantly being moved about within the space, and therefore even without having to think about the exercises, the patient is doing them in her daily life. There is also the feeling that muscle has so much nutrition and defence against infection that placing the implant in this location has a better chance if infection is felt to be a cause.

However, even placement under the muscle results in more than occasional contractures, so the search for a reliable solution continued. An implant with the same silicone rubber shell and silicone gel content, but with a foam (polyurethane) covering was developed, and this seemed reliably to reduce the contracture rate to 1% or less for the first five to seven years after surgery, but concerns were raised about the long term health risks of the foam as the body digested it, and the product (Meme, or Replicon) was withdrawn from the market in 1991. In the theory that it was the rough surface of the foam-covered implant that reduced the contracture rate, a textured or rough surface silicone rubber shell implant was developed, and is widely used in the USA, although it has only very recently been approved for use in Canada. This implant has met with some success over the past five or so years, although opinions vary as to how reliably it results in soft breasts, and there are other problems with their use.

THE SILICONE SCARE

This is a difficult topic to discuss in a non-technical fashion, while dealing effectively with the facts as we know them.

Silicone gel filled implants were taken off the market except for investigational purposes in 1992 by the US Food and Drug Administration and Canada's parallel body, the Health Protection Branch, soon followed with a similar ruling.

There were several concerns which prompted these rulings: possible risk of cancer, a possible link to immune related diseases, and leakage of the implants.

We know that breast cancer occurs in about one out of every nine women in North America today. Some women with breast implants, therefore, are bound to develop breast cancer. However, large numbers (many thousands) of patients have been followed for long periods, especially in studies done at the University of Calgary, and it seems quite clear that implants do not increase the risk of a woman developing breast cancer, nor do they result in significant compromises in its treatment, when it is found. Implants do make mammograms somewhat less accurate, although saline-filled implants are better than were the gel filled implants.

Connective tissue diseases are illnesses, the most common of which is rheumatoid arthritis, in which the body's immune system reacts to parts of the body, causing symptoms. In arthritis, these symptoms are mainly in the joints, but may also involve other body systems. In a small number of patients with breast implants, symptoms of allergic or immune illness have been seen, such as scleroderma or other diseases. Scleroderma is a disease which causes hardening and thickening of the skin and other organs, caused by fibrous tissue ingrowth. We expect to see approximately 2% of all women developing these symptoms, so it is not surprising that some patients with implants will develop similar symptoms, but not caused by the implants. Since the ban on gel-filled implants, research has continued to show the unlikelihood of a link between the implants and these types of illnesses. However, these conclusions are based on statistics, and it remains possible, although unlikely, that a very small number of patients develop immune related illness from implants. Scleroderma seems to be most common in Japan, where liquid silicone for injection is still used for procedures such as breast augmentation. Liquid silicone is chemically different from silicone gel. Furthermore, since it is not bound by a capsule, there is more risk that it will migrate into undesirable locations.

The third concern relates to leakage of the implants. Careful study, especially from the University of Toronto, has shown that gel filled implants leak much earlier and at a much higher rate than was previously thought. Implants used between approximately 1972 and 1987, depending on the manufacturer, may develop small or major leaks as early as four or five years after surgery. The main reason the implants were taken off the market by the FDA was that Dow Corning knew there was a higher risk of leakage than they told plastic surgeons.

On the other hand, the presence of a leak does not seem to cause illness, nor does it seem to cause very significant silicone amounts to circulate elsewhere in the body.

The diagnosis of leaking, gel-filled implants is difficult, and, from the information now available, it seems that the best course, if a patient has older implants (pre-1987, especially), is that they be removed and replaced with saline implants.

MAMMOGRAMS

Routine pre-operative mammograms are recommended for patients who are thirty-five or older. After surgery, the usual recommendation is for a mammogram every year after forty years of age.

Saline implants placed under the muscle give a better mammogram picture than what was possible with silicone gel-filled implants, but an extra view done by the mammographer is advised to achieve about 85% of the accuracy achieved in patients without implants.

ALTERNATIVE FILL SUBSTANCES

Research continues in the attempt to find a more ideal implant. To try to make rippling less of a problem, and to make mammograms more accurate, soy oil filled implants have been tried. This research, however, is in a preliminary stage. I think there is no safer filler than saline, and extensive long term testing is needed to develop a reliable, and safe substitute. Because the human body is 71% salt water, if a saline filled implant leaks, the saline goes into your general circulation and results in no ill effects, other than loss of breast fullness.

SIZE

Historically there were many methods used to determine breast implant size, but these were, surprisingly, usually dependent on the surgeon's sense of balance and esthetics. I have modified a method first described in the early 1980's by a Canadian surgeon practising in the Los Angeles area, along with information I have learned from surgeons in Texas and the eastern USA. First, we ask the patient to buy a bra of the size she wants to be, and to buy it by trying bras on wearing a sheer blouse or T-shirt, stuffing the bra cup with tissue of other fillers. She then comes in to the office and we have her put the bra on and place a device in the bra. The device is a temporary type of implant which can be filled with water until the bra cup is filled to the desired volume with implant plus her own breast. At this point, I examine the dimensions of the patient's chest, and if she has sufficient space on her

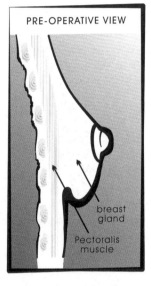

9c)

Pre-operative view (cross section)

The breast after augmentation. The implant may be placed under the breast gland (d), or under the breast gland and the pectoralis muscle (e).

9d)

9e)

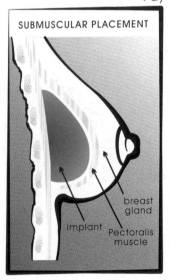

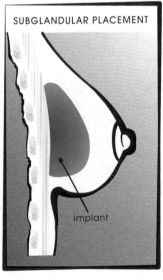

chest to allow the placement of an implant of the size she desires (which is usually the case), we simply use that size of prosthesis. Adjustments can be made for differences in size between the two sides. Most important, the patient determines the size, with my help.

INCISIONS, PLACEMENT LOCATION

Three incision locations are possible, and our main aim is to keep the scar as inconspicuous as possible, while maintaining patient safety and excellent results. The most commonly used choices are either at the edge of the areola or under the breast, while occasionally we use an incision in the armpit. The incision under the breast offers the easiest procedure but in some patients, especially with skin more prone to form thicker scars (patients with darker skin types, especially), is inadvisable. The incision at the edge of the areola usually results in a good scar, but some patients find this location objectionable for esthetic or emotional reasons. When I use this approach I usually tunnel down between the skin and the breast until the bottom of the gland is reached before coming back up under the gland, so as not to interfere with the nipple and the ducts leading from the breast gland. The armpit approach has been less popular with surgeons because there have been problems with positioning the implant correctly once the space has been created for it, but these problems are now being overcome with newer technology, and the use of endo-scopic surgery, which offers us a more reliable way to do this technique.

The implant can be located either above or below the pectoral muscle. Placing the implant above the muscle is feasible in women who have a moderate A-cup breast or larger, can be done under local anaesthetic with sedation (twilight anaesthesia), and allows the patient to return to her usual activities a little faster than below the muscle. Many surgeons also believe it gives a good appearance earlier than the sub-muscular placement.

The under muscle (sub-muscular) placement offers a possible advantage of lower contracture rates, and in very small breasted women, saline implants will have a risk of appearing rippling or wavey with movement if they are placed directly under the skin and small gland. In most patients, I advise a sub-muscular placement, for these reasons, although this approach requires a general anaesthetic, results in slightly more post-operative pain, and takes a little longer to achieve the final esthetic result.

POST-OP

I usually see patients the first working day after surgery and check carefully for any problems, discuss how they are feeling, and review any concerns she may have. Stitches are removed a few days later and the exercises to keep the implant soft and mobile are reviewed. Barring any problems or concerns, we usually have another visit six weeks later and at six months, and then annually if possible.

BREAST FEEDING

There is usually no interference with the function of the breast gland, and as long as there is some sensation to the nipple (it is rare for complete loss of sensation to occur) nursing is possible. However, not all new mothers are successful at nursing even without implants, so no guarantees can be made.

BREAST LIFT

The natural shape of the breast gradually changes with time. Some women become dissatisfied with the shape of their breasts due to droop and wish to restore or even improve upon their youthful shape.

To understand breast lift surgery, the development and anatomy of the breast must be understood. Surgery has very definite limits and only turns back the clock rather than stopping it.

ANATOMY

The breast is a skin gland, related closely to sweat glands, but specialized to the production of milk. It develops at puberty, from the small gland button which exists under the nipple at birth. As the gland grows, the surrounding fat grows, and the overlying skin expands. Initially, this gives a cone shaped breast with the nipple at the peak, but very quickly, the skin continues to expand under the weight of the gland and a relatively tear-drop shape develops.

With pregnancy and nursing, further changes occur. The gland enlarges rapidly, putting (sometimes painful) stretch on the skin and underlying tissues; often this is great enough and rapid enough to cause damage to the elastic fibres of the skin (causing stretch marks). Later, the gland shrinks to its original size or may be significantly smaller, leaving an expanded skin covering.

We think of the breast as a gland which is supported by the

brassiere-like overlying skin. As the skin is expanded, or the gland shrinks, or both occur, the gland drops to the bottom of the bra (skin envelope).

The breast is only loosely attached to the underlying chest (pectoral) muscle, and exercises to tighten the breast have little or no benefit. This is disappointing to patients, and often they come in having tried everything prior to a surgical consultation.

Generally, the degree of drooping is described by how far the breast and the nipple / areola have dropped below the level of the fold under the breast. Some patients feel they have developed drooping but the nipple and areola are still above the level of the fold; in this type of case, the cause is generally loss of breast volume alone and placement of an implant is the usual recommended treatment. In most cases when the patient complains of drooping, the nipple and areola have descended below the level of the fold, and the degree of droop is described by the plastic surgeon in terms of the distance from the level of the fold to the level of the nipple. Mild droop is within one centimetre of the fold, moderate from one to two centimeters and more severe drooping is when the nipple / areola is three centimeters or more below the level of the fold.

TECHNICAL DETAILS

The surgeon must reduce the size of the "skin-brassiere," increase the size of the gland, or do a procedure which in some way combines both. Furthermore, the shape of the breast is a complex, three dimensional one, and a successful lift requires a three dimensional approach to re-shaping.

Many procedures have been devised to try to reduce the surgical scars resulting from lifts. The traditional techniques involve removing skin in vertical and horizontal dimensions below and around the nipple and areola, and moving the nipple areolar complex up to a predetermined level. The surgeon usually starts by marking

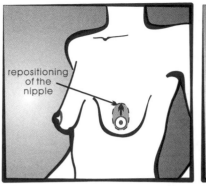 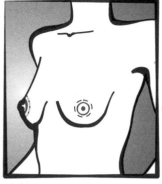

repositioning
of the
nipple

10a)   10b)

With mild droop or a small breast, it may be possible to limit incisions to just around the areola.

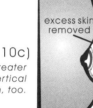

10c)

A larger gland and/or greater droop may require a vertical incision, too.

excess skin
removed

In some cases, however, a formal skin tightening horizontally and vertically is needed.

10d)   10e)

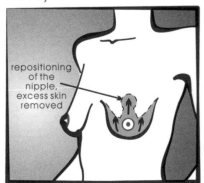 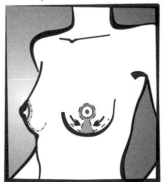

repositioning
of the
nipple,
excess skin
removed

101

the skin with a surgical marking pen, with the patient awake and either sitting or standing. These marks are used to guide incisions and nipple placement during the operation when the patient is lying down and dimensions are distorted. Often, the patient is sat up during the operation while under anesthesia, to check the accuracy of nipple placement before the completion of surgery.

The extent of the incisions will depend on the degree of drooping and the technique employed. Usually, if the patient is having a breast lift only, mild droop can be treated by removing a doughnut of skin from around the areola, and tightening the skin concentrically (like a purse-string) around the areola. More significant degrees of droop require a vertical incision, and major drooping may involve a horizontal incision which is concealed as much as possible in the fold.

RECENT INNOVATIONS

Because the treatment of moderate to severe degrees of drooping has traditionally involved extensive incisions, creating scars which are prominent and symptomatic for prolonged periods, efforts have been directed towards reducing the length of incisions, while trying to maintain the three dimensional effective lift of traditional techniques. This has met with varying success, depending on the size of the breasts being lifted, and the quality of the patient's skin. In Europe, where nude sun-bathing is common, and small breasts are viewed as desirable, short scar techniques for breast lift and reduction are common, but so are drastic breast reductions and reductions in what North Americans would often view as normal or smallish breasts. North American women are more concerned with the quality of scars, and the overall shape of the breast, and short scar techniques, while used, have not been applied quite as universally as they have in Europe.

I usually try to restrict the length of the scars under the breast as much as is possible, and in some cases this incision can be eliminated entirely. In minor degrees of droop, a doughnut lift may be enough; however, in practice, this usually occurs when I am doing a volume increase (augmentation) at the same time.

For many patients, because the droop has occurred simultaneously with significant loss of breast size, an augmentation is desirable. Fullness of the upper half of the breast can usually only be achieved and maintained with the placement of an implant, and the longevity of a breast lift is definitely increased by the use of implants. However, augmentation mammaplasty may be either undesirable to the patient or the patient may be satisfied with her breast size.

RISKS & POSSIBLE COMPLICATIONS

As with any surgical procedure, breast lift can result in infection, bleeding, and delayed healing. The risk of these occurring is quite small. Generally, the risk of infection in clean, elective surgical procedures is about 1%, and that of significant post-operative bleeding is about the same. If we are careful to avoid operating on patients with untreated high blood pressure, or those taking blood thinning medications including anti-inflammatories like aspirin, the risk of bleeding is probably even less. Massive bleeding requiring transfusion is exceedingly rare, and few plastic surgeons have had such cases for lift procedures alone. Even in breast reduction, a somewhat similar operation, transfusion has become quite unusual.

The blood supply to the nipple can be compromised in a lift, resulting in partial or even complete loss of the nipple, but this complication, which is unusual in breast reduction, is extremely rare in lift procedures. Similarly, loss of feeling to the nipple is less common in lifts than in either augmention or reduction mammaplasty.

However, asymmetry, and modest degrees of unsatifactory shape are more common, and drooping gradually or, occasionally rapidly, recurrs. Skin with poor tone and elasticity prior to the surgery will be more prone to recurrence than thicker, more elastic skin. Most women with significant drooping have either thin and poorly elastic skin to begin with, or went through pronounced engorgement and enlargment with pregancy. In the former type of patient, she must be satisfied with more modest results of the operation and must understand that some early recurrence will occur.

The most difficult complication of breast lift surgery to treat, however, is related to the height of the nipple-areolar complex. If it is sited too high, it will be difficult for the patient to wear low cut clothing, and brasierres and bathing suits will similarly be awkward. Generally, if this occurs, the best treatment is to wait until the skin below the nipple stretches and then to tighten this with a horizontal tightening, which will effectively lower the nipple and areola. Similarly, asymmetry is best treated after a cautious period of waiting.

SUCTION LIPOPLASTY

If you have troublesome localized fat tissue that is unresponsive to diet or exercise, suction assisted removal may be an extremely valuable procedure and deserves your consideration.

INTRODUCTION

A method of fat tissue removal is available for selected use for a variety of conditions. Any individual contemplating this type of treatment will, of course, require a personal examination and consultation. Determining whether or not you are a suitable candidate for this procedure will be based on a variety of factors. Each individual must be examined carefully to determine what may be best in his or her own case.

FUNDAMENTAL CONSIDERATIONS

For the most part, the size and shape of our bodies are characteristics inherited from our parents. The degree to which these characteristics are manifest depends to a certain extent on our calorie intake and our energy expenditure but the basic body shape is an inherited trait.

To understand the potential of suction lipoplasty, several additional facts should be known. First, you should be aware that we all have a definite number of fat cells. There is evidence to show that an increased number of fat cells is associated with early over-feeding. Because of this, weight gain and loss is dependent more on how much fat is present in the individual cells than in the number of cells. The removal of, or destruction of, cells will largely prevent the fat from re-accumulating in those areas treated.

HISTORY

Surgical removal of excess fat tissue has been performed for almost 100 years. However, until recently, the methods used required surface incisions and incision closures that did not usually leave minor scars. There was always a serious question as to whether the final results, in terms of permanent scarring, justified the procedures.

In the 1970's, a French surgeon, working in Paris, developed a technique using a blunt tipped, hollow metal tube along with a high vacuum suction to remove fat tissue in a number of different body locations. This method became widely used and found wide acceptance by both surgeons and patients. Recent refinements have made the surgery safer, less painful, and produce even better results.

TECHNICAL DETAILS

Removal of excess fat tissue is accomplished by inserting a narrow metal tube through a small skin incision and applying suction. The tube has a round end and one or several openings along the side close to the tip. As suction is applied, it draws the fat globules into the tube. Passing the instrument forward and backwards shears off the fat tissue particles which pass into the tube and are thus removed .

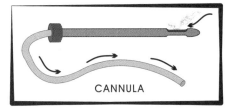

A hollow tube (cannula) with openings near the end, is inserted through the skin. Suction is applied, either with a machine or a syringe.

11a)

CANNULA

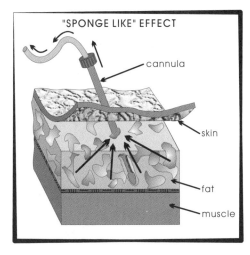

"SPONGE LIKE" EFFECT

cannula

skin

fat

muscle

11b)

The cannula is passed back and forth through the fat, creating a network of tunnels and spaces, and reducing the fat.

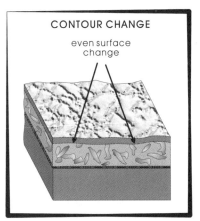

CONTOUR CHANGE

even surface change

11c)

As the spaces collapse, the overlying skin shrinks to fit the reduced volume.

107

As shown in the accompanying diagram, the basic technique is the removal of fat globules in what can be described as a multiple tunnel fashion, essentially creating a "sponge-like" effect within the tissues. By developing the numerous interconnecting and closely related spaces, the fullness, firmness and size of the area is reduced. Ultimately, there is collapse or shrinkage in the treated area, with a secondary surface contour change.

Leaving small areas of tissue intact between the tunnels preserves the larger blood vessels and nerves that nourish the overlying skin. By removing all the fat tissue and creating one large cavity, one would indeed create greater shrinkage, but it would also reduce the normal blood circulation to the skin. This would result in loss of skin and scarring, infection and deformity.

The object is not to remove all the fat tissue. A layer must be preserved to avoid undesirable effects. This layer can be thinner in some areas of the body than others.

An important factor in determining any final result is the degree of normal skin elasticity. The skin of younger individuals is more favorable than that of older individuals and results in even shrinkage and a smoother final surface.

In older skin this elastic quality is diminished and it is possible that some wrinkling or irregularity will remain following procedure, even under the best of circumstances. If elasticity is felt to be inadequate to give a good esthetic result, you may be advised to have a skin tightening operation of the treated areas, alone, or in combination with suction. This is most common in the abdomen (tummy tucks) but is also useful in the neck, the buttocks and thighs.

New Modifications:

a)   The "Syringe Method"
        Initially, suction was done by connecting to a powerful vacuum machine. For the past few years, simply

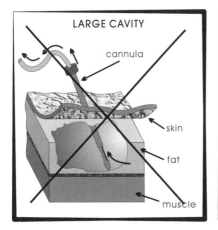

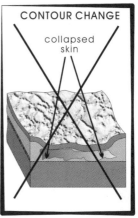

11d)   11e)

We do not remove all the fat. This would create a large space. The skin would shrink irregularly and create a deformity.

using a large syringe which is locked open has resulted in less trauma to small blood vessels and better control of the amount removed. I routinely use this method.

b)   The "Tumescent Technique"
        By injecting large quantities of a solution containing very diluted local anaesthetic, adrenaline and salt water, bleeding is reduced, less bruising results, and it may even be possible to do the surgery under local (awake) anaesthesia.

c)   Small Diameter Cannulae
        By using smaller suction tubes, more precision has been obtained, and there is less trauma, less bleeding with less bruising.

d)   Ultrasonic assisted Liposuction (UAL)

        This newer, still experimental technique, was developed in Italy and Israel; it uses ultrasonic energy to liquify the fat first, then gentle suction to remove the fat. The advantages are said to be that it requires less effort for the surgeon; is supposed to result in less bleeding, allowing the removal of larger quantities of fat; and more easily removes fat in areas where there is a lot of tough fibrous tissue, such as in male breast development, and deep in the lower back of men. However, the tube requires constant cooling with salt water and must be kept moving, or serious burns can result. A task force to study the technique and determine its safety has been set up by the American Society of Plastic and Reconstructive Surgeons in order to determine whether the equipment should be approved for general use by the FDA in the U.S.A. Many who have used the technique do not believe it reduces bleeding significantly, and, therefore, feel it offers little advantage to patients, and carries a higher risk and cost. However, the technology is still evolving.

CELLULITE

The term "cellulite" is used to describe a particular appearance of the skin and underlying fat but is blamed on a special kind of fat for which a variety of treatments are recommended by non-surgical personnel.

Detailed microscopic examination of these areas does not reveal any difference in the fat cells as compared to the fat cells in non-cellulite areas. The term cellulite, therefore, refers to the bumpy or wavy condition of the skin and is probably due to tethering of the skin through the fat to the underlying muscle by some strong fibres and bulging of the fat cells between. The bulging is irregular and, therefore, gives the skin an irregular surface contour. The skin is loose and sagging but remains attached tightly at the fibre attachments, leaving indentations. The only way to significantly treat the so-called cellulite is to tighten the skin by traditional techniques, employing long incisions, such as a buttock/thigh lift (see Body Contour Surgery chapter).

A patient for suction lipectomy should anticipate that the same limitations exist in cellulite cases as in other circum-stances where lack of elasticity is prominent. The fibres which tether the skin to the underlying muscles cannot be broken down by laser treatment, vibration massage or by other forms of non-medical therapy and one should be aware of the limitations of all treatments for this.

However, it is possible to treat the most prominent dimples and indentations by dividing some of the tethering fibres and injecting a small quantity of fat to prevent re-adherence. This is very time consuming and may bring mixed results.

RISKS, POTENTIAL COMPLICATIONS AND NORMAL POST-SURGICAL EVENTS

Now that you understand some of the mechanics of the surgical suction lipectomy, the risks as well as the normal course of events following this operation should be more easily understood.

To begin with, this treatment is for localized fat deposits only. It is not for general obesity. The quantity limitations for fat tissue removal at any one procedure use to be approximately 2,000 cc. (1,000 cc. is approximately equal to one quart of combined fat tissue and blood components), but with recent innovations in technique such as the use of the tumescent method, this maximum has been revised upward significantly. Removal of excessive amounts might require a blood transfusion. For this reason it is undesirable. Approximately 20-25% of the material removed use to consist of blood products and 75-80% actual fat tissue. Using the tumescent solution, the proportion which is blood products is very much less. In fact, we see the fat removal as being nearly pure, but there is still some loss of blood under the skin after completion of surgery, so some caution is still justified. Presently, in my practice, we do not go beyond about 4,500cc, or ten pounds.

This represents a significant reduction and amounts up to this can be removed on an ambulatory, or outpatient, basis.

111

SCARS

There will always be a skin mark at the site where the surface incision is made. This varies in length from 1/4 inch to 1/2 inch but we try to place it in an area where it is inconspicuous.

Bruising of the treated area must be expected although it is variable in degree and sometimes quite extensive. There is no way of avoiding this. A compression garment, like a girdle with zippers and velcro, is used according to the individual requirements. Provision is be made for voiding functions so that the garment need not be removed during the first few days after surgery.

Bruising usually lasts from 7 to 10 days and sometimes even longer. The compression dressing is a very important part of the procedure. We now have also added an adhesive-backed foam product to our dressing for the first few days and this has also resulted in less bruising.

Since most of the fat cells are removed and some simply disrupted, a fair amount of drainage from the surgical site should also be expected.

Depending upon the location, your pre-operative skin tone, and the amount of fat tissue removed, some irregularity or waviness of the surface may also occur. Since the final surface contour depends on the collapse of the fat tissue later, after the tunnels are made, it is surprising that surface irregularity is not a more notable condition afterwards. When there is good skin tension and the fat tissue removal is quite regular, the surface remains remarkably smooth.

There is a relatively narrow margin between removal of sufficient tissue and removal of too much tissue. Therefore, we are conservative in our removals if there is any question as it is easier to remove further tissue at the smaller second sitting than to try to replace fat for a significant contour deformity.

Other potential problems include adverse surface pigmentation and dimpling at the places where the underside of the skin may adhere to the tissues, extensive bruising, and some permanent sensory loss which is usually limited. Occasionally, there will be discomfort and localized burning sensations during the healing period.

Final contour and shrinkage are probably not reached for at least 6-9 months, but significant change is obvious only days after surgery, as the initial swelling begins to resolve.

I usually do the surgery under general anesthesia. In certain cases, we do it under local anaesthesia or a local with sedation, but this is not appropriate for every patient.

Occasionally, the post-operative appearance does not look remarkably different than it did before the surgery. This is the result of swelling within the tissue and it may take several weeks or months to change. Premature conclusions are therefore unwarranted. Patience is required and rewarded.

Areas for Suction Lipectomy Include:

Chin & Neck (alone or with a facelift)
Breast reduction (may be used to reduce the fullness at the side of the breast)
Accessory breast folds
Male breast reduction
Abdomen (this procedure may be used alone or in combination with abdominal surgery for removal of redundant skin folds)
Waist ("love handles")
Hips
Thighs (saddlebag deformity) -- the most frequent area for treatment that responds remarkably well in selected situations
Thighs (inner and upper thighs). Used alone or in combination with surgical excision
Knees (reduction of prominent inner surfaces as well as fullness above or below)
Ankles and lower legs

Others (fat accumulations in other localized areas apart from those already mentioned)

Your personal attitude is also important in determining whether or not you are a good candidate for this procedure. Unreasonable expectations can be a source of disappointment. With a realistic attitude and a clear idea of the aims of surgery, the results can be both dramatic and very satisfying, which is why suction lipoplasty has become so popular since its introduction.

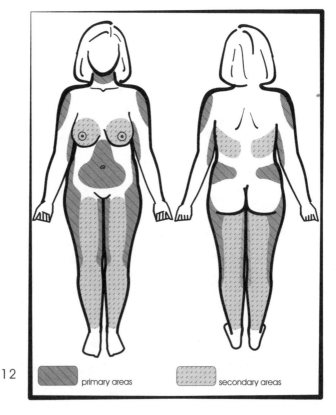

12

primary areas   secondary areas

Common (primary), and less common (secondary) areas treated by suction lipoplasty.

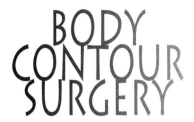

BODY CONTOUR SURGERY

Despite the great advances which have been achieved since the advent of suction lipoplasty, surgeons and patients are still unable to restore skin elasticity. When weight gain and loss, age, pregnancy and disease cause skin to be loose, more traditional surgical techniques must still be used to tighten skin and re-contour it to the underlying shape. Just as when an individual loses several inches around their waist, clothing must be altered by "taking it in" or removing a dart, in other locations, the skin, which is like the fabric covering the underlying body, must be altered by removal of excess.

By body contour surgery, we usually refer to suction assisted lipoplasty plus procedures such as abdominoplasty, thigh lifts, and upper arm tightening surgery. Suction assisted lipoplasty has been previously discussed, but may be used to complement the other, more traditional body contouring procedures.

The most common body contouring operation, aside from liposuction, is abdominoplasty, or the Tummy Tuck, as it is commonly referred to by lay persons. Though there are been mini-operations for the abdomen which have become possible since the advent of liposuction, in the average patient, who comes with skin laxity and some fat accumulations in the abdomen, flanks and other regions after one or more pregnancies or previous surgical

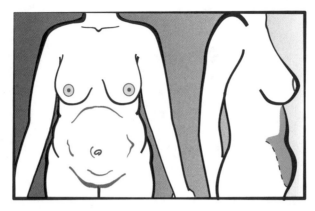

13a)

In abdominoplasty, there may be loose, sagging skin, lax muscles, fat accumulations, and a high or low belly button.

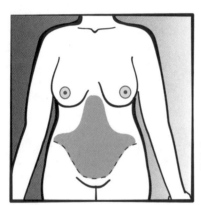

An incision is made in or just above the pubic area. Skin in the shaded area is separated from the underlying muscles.

13b)

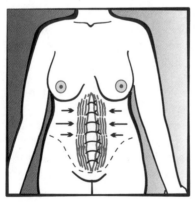

The abdominal muscles are tightened with stitches.

13c)

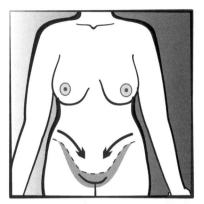

13d)

Abdominal skin is drawn downward and in from the flanks. A small opening is made for the belly button.

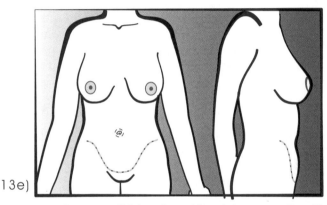

13e)

A more youthful contour of the abdomen results, with scars hidden within the bikini line.

procedures, a full abdominoplasty with a lengthy incision is required. In fact, the most common form of abdominoplasty which I currently use is not a lesser variation of a traditional procedure, but is, instead, more extensive, because so much more is known about how to achieve the best results.

Buttock and thigh lifts are done via incisions which are placed along the panty or Bikini line through the hip and low back region for the outer thigh and buttock, and high up the inner thigh at its junction with the groin for the inner thigh. These operations are similar in concept to the abdominoplasty, but are less commonly done.

HISTORY

Removal of a fold of skin plus the underlying fat dates back to the early part of the 20th century. In the 1960's, the operation was refined considerably and popularized by a Brazilian surgeon, Pitanguy. He also did early thigh and buttock lifts. Many of his improvements are with us to this day. Further advances were made, particularly in incision design, by a Quebec surgeon, Paule Regnault, who also worked on innovations in breast lift and reduction surgery. However, the two most significant advances in the last quarter century have been the advent of suction lipoplasty, which allowed for treatment of the abdomen fat, with or without skin removal, and the deep layer support techniques of Dr. T. Lockwood of Kansas City. He carefully looked at the anatomy of the abdominal wall, and decided that there was merit in using the superficial fascia, a layer of thin but strong tissue, part way down in the fat layer, as the main means of support, in repairing the skin incisions during both abdominoplasties and thigh lift procedures. This layer had been known to surgeons and anatomists for many years, but most plastic surgeons never felt it had enough strength to be of significant use in repairing the abdominal wall and it was often either ignored or only loosely stitched.

Patients for buttock and thigh lift may initially come to their consultation requesting liposuction, complaining of unsightly fat and "cellulite" but, because of laxity of the skin and deep tissues, should be told that the results of suction alone may be quite disappointing. While suction offers an operation with little in the way of post-op scars, it will result in further loss of skin tone and likely significant contour irregularities. For this reason they should be offered a lift procedure which, despite the significant scar, will result in a much restored appearance to the thigh and buttock. Some of these patients will have had suction done in the past and wish to have something further done. The situation is similar to patients who have had only suction done in the neck and have residual neck skin and muscle redundancy for which the only treatment is a face and necklift.

The usual patient presenting for abdominoplasty has had previous pregnancies, and has usually decided not to have any more children. (Future pregnancies will tend to re-stretch the skin and may cause recurrence of the shape the patient feels is unsatisfactory). She may or may not have had Caesarean sections, or other abdominal surgery. The low gynecologic and Caesarean scar (called a Pfannenstiel incision by gynecologists) often is adherent to the underlying muscle, and above the incision, the non-adherent abdominal skin and fat often droop, and fold over the site of the incision. In some cases, with skin lying against skin, there may be so much problem with moisture causing skin irritation, that the medical insurance will pay for a procedure to reduce the overhanging skin, but a formal, cosmetic abdominoplasty will usually require patient payment.

The vertical abdominal muscles (the rectus abdominis) have often been stretched, and they may be separated down the midline, giving bulging of the central abdomen, and in more severe cases, there may even be a hernia of the belly button (umbilicus). In a hernia, not only does the abdomen bulge, but some of the contents of the abdominal cavity (internal organs, fat, etc.) may bulge through a weak part of the abdominal wall. Other old surgical scars may further distort the shape of the abdomen.

Occasionally, I also have male patients who want abdominoplasty surgery. Men often carry most of their trunk fat inside the abdominal cavity, rather than under the skin, and abdominoplasty is somewhat less effective at reducing and recontouring in men. Yet, they will usually have a reasonable and satisfying result.

In patients with less dramatic changes, a modified, or

mini-abdominoplasty is effective. In this procedure, there is less excess skin and a significant amount of fat, so the major procedure is liposuction with the addition of a smaller skin tightening procedure. At one time, about three quarters of my patients seemed to fall into this category; the reverse is now true. This is because I feel I must do a full abdominoplasty in most of my patients to give them the result they have envisaged for themselves; a lesser operation leaves them somewhat disappointed.

TECHNICAL DETAILS

The goal of these procedures is to achieve a youthful contour to the abdomen and flanks, both at rest and with activity. Because photographs are taken with patients in static, or unmoving poses, a result from liposuction which looks good with the flash lighting and stationary pose of medical photography, may in fact be less than ideal in real life. Dimpling and irregularities of the skin may be quite mild in a young patient who has good skin tone and no children carried through a full pregnancy. In an older individual or one who has less tone after weight loss, pregnancy or illness, there may substantial skin tone reduction.

Therefore, the operation removes excess skin, tightens the underlying muscles and repairs a hernia if it is present, and positions the incision along a line which, if carefully planned, can lie concealed within the lines of a bathing suit. The belly button is separated from the surrounding skin, and usually all the skin and fat below the level of the belly button can be removed so that the skin around the belly button is at the level of the pubis, and skin from higher up is tightened and brought down to the belly button level when the operation is completed. The belly button is brought through a new hole at an appropriate level and stitched to the surrounding skin. With experience, the surgeon can usually create an abdominal contour which is not only tighter, but natural looking as well.

Less commonly, patients request treatment for redundant skin and fat in the arms. This is particularly a problem after weight loss, but may be a concern with increasing age and fat accumulation combined with a familial tendency to such shape. Brachioplasty is the term used for re-forming the arm, and this, once again, can be done by

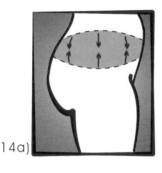

14a)

In a buttock / outer thigh lift, skin is drawn from the flanks and up from the areas to be lifted.

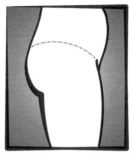

14b)

The incision is carefully planned so resulting scars can be concealed in bikini lines.

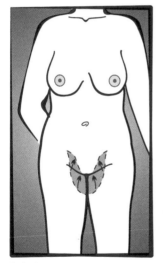

14c)

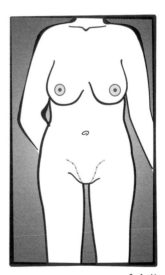

14d)

In an inner thigh lift, the bikini line incisions are along the groin and pubic-thigh creases to lift and tighten the upper inner thigh. Inner and outer thigh lifts are combined in a Lower Body Lift.

means of suction alone, in appropriate patients, or in combination with skin tightening surgery. The challenge here is to place the incision in a location which is stable and does not migrate into a prominent position as healing occurs.

RISKS AND POSSIBLE COMPLICATIONS

Abdominoplasty, and the related body contouring operations, all share similar risks and possible complications. Like all surgical procedures, bleeding or infection can occur, although both are unusual. If they do occur, they may require surgical treatment, hospitalization, or may be managed with lesser measures in some cases. Infection, when diagnosed early and not severe, may respond to antibiotics by mouth, for example.

Because a space exists between the muscles of the abdominal wall and the overlying skin and fat, fluid can accumulate during the early healing phase, until these layers re-unite. For this reason, we use a drain, a soft tube with multiple holes which is placed between the skin and the muscle and exits to a small plastic bottle and removes the fluid (serum) which your body produces during the healing phase. This is removed at five to seven days after surgery. Occasionally, serum will continue to accumulate and collect, forming a seroma, which is like a lake of serum under the surface. This sometimes requires removal, either with a needle or with a new placement of a drain, but this is only a temporary problem, and usually resolve gradually.

However, problems with poor or delayed healing of the incision can occur, leaving areas with widened scars after crust formation. This is a much greater risk in smokers, so avoidance of smoking is essential.

Formation of blood clots in the legs (thrombophlebitis), with possible passage of a clot to the lung can occur with any of these procedures. While rare, this is potentially a very serious problem. At one time, abdominoplasty patients were routinely kept on bed rest for several days after surgery; today, patients are routinely up and walking within a day or so after surgery. Early mobilization has always been felt to be one of the best preventive measures against thrombophlebitis, and we believe it to be of value in body contour surgery.

MALE ESTHETIC SURGERY

Although reports, in the late 1980's, that men were rapidly embracing esthetic surgery were probably exaggerated, the number of men seeking esthetic surgery is gradually and steadily increasing.

There are areas of esthetic surgery which vary a little or not at all between gender, procedures that vary more so, and some that are particular to men. In facelift surgery, for example, there are small nuances of the execution of surgery which make the difference between a good and an excellent result, such as the placement of incisions according to the hair distribution and the shape of the sideburns. In eyelid and brow surgery, the esthetic shape desired is different in men than in women; a lower brow and fuller eyelid is masculine and feminizing of the eye region is undesirable. The shape of an attractive male nose is different from that of a beautiful female nose, but there, as with any rhinoplasty surgery, it is most important to listen to the desires of the individual patient, and it is important for the patient to try to express those desires as clearly as possible.

The main areas which are particular to male esthetic surgery, however, are in the treatment of male pattern baldness, male body contour surgery including lipoplasty, and the recently developed methods for augmenting the penis.

MALE PATTERN BALDNESS

Surgery for the treatment of baldness, or alopecia, has progressed significantly since the days when the transplanted plugs looked like corn rows. Simultaneously, there is better understanding of male pattern baldness, and how it is best treated.

It is well known that the tendency to develop baldness is inherited from the mother's side, and that this tendency may or may not be expressed or come out, in any individual.

Usually, if an individual is going to develop substantial hair loss, there is already some thinning beginning in the early twenties, and this may follow one of several patterns.

Treatment may be medical and surgical. There has been some benefit from the use of minoxidil, marketed as Rogaine, a drug which was initially used as a treatment for high blood pressure but found to have a side effect of reducing baldness in some patients. It is used topically, as a solution which is applied with accessories from a bottle. Response to minoxidil is variable, and it must be used indefinitely in order to maintain its effects.

Surgery may involve reducing the bald area by means of scalp reduction; expanding the hair bearing region with tissue expanders which are temporary, inflatable silicone implants which are first implanted, then gradually filled with saline solution over a period of weeks to months, and then removed after the overlying scalp has been expanded to a surface area which will fill the desired area required; and hair grafts, which now consist of clusters of only a few hairs or even single hairs to give a more natural result. The exact surgical plan depends on the pattern of hair loss because this determines what reconstructive options are available. Usually, the treatment must involve staged procedures over time in order to give the optimal result, and this is ideally begun once hair loss has slowed, or stabilized. The methods used also vary according to the personal preferences of the surgeon.

MALE BODY CONTOUR SURGERY

Although much of the field of body contour surgery is the same in men as in women, certain points are relevant.

Fat accumulation is quite different in men than in women, and obesity is unfortunately less treatable by lipoplasty. Women tend to accumulate fat on the outside of the body, beneath the skin but outside the muscles and internal organs. Men, on the other hand, accumulate a great proportion of their fat inside the body, around the internal organs, and at a level inaccessible to suction lipoplasty.

This does not mean there is no application of suction in men, but it does mean that the expected result from suction of the abdomen is different from that in women. Men tend to have definite fat deposits in the flanks and above the buttocks in the back, the so-called love-handles, and these are generally well treated by suction. In some men, there may be substantial improvement in abdominal contour with suction.

Male breast development, or gynecomastia is a common problem which begins in teenage years and often persists into adulthood. It may be associated with mild adolescent obesity or may be seen in otherwise complete normal individuals. The current popularity of anabolic steroids in body builders is possibly associated with an increase in gynecomastia.

Depending on how much the breasts have developed, treatment may consist of simple removal of the gland through a small incision at the edge of the areola, suction of the surrounding fat and removal of the gland, or, in cases where the gland has grown so much as to cause the breast to take on a female shape with stretching of the over lying skin envelope, may involve a skin reduction procedure with incisions similar to those of the various degrees of breast lifts. Most cases are handled relatively simply, and efforts are being directed towards developing suction techniques which may allow the entire gland to be removed by suction alone.

Generally, excision of male breast tissue, with or without suction lipoplasty of the chest, can be carried out on an ambulatory basis with little difficulty. Serious complications are unusual, and the risks are similar to those of other body contouring procedures, and include infection, bleeding, and sensory changes. The removal of the breast gland can also occasionally result in the nipple and areola becoming sunken, so generally an attempt is made to prevent this by leaving a thin layer of underlying breast tissue beneath it. Occasionally, there can be a recurrence of the breast tissue enlargement.

PENIS ENHANCEMENT SURGERY

Enlargement of the penis is a new field of esthetic surgery and is not currently being done by most plastic surgeons. Some attempts at enhancing the penis size have resulted in significant problems and generated controversy due to serious complications and, perhaps, unethical practices. However, a few individuals are attempting to do responsible surgery and carefully assess their results in a manner which will allow them and their peers to determine whether this kind of surgery should be offered to the public and how it should be done. A fairly large number of patients has been treated by several methods and, when done by the right surgeon for the right reasons, the surgery seems to offer some significant change reasonably safely.

The results could not be properly evaluated until some idea of what the objectives of surgery could be established, and this meant establishing what was considered to be normal penis size. It was not surprising, but was rather humorous, to have a large gathering of esthetic surgeons told, in a lecture given by Dr. R. Stubbs at the Canadian Society of Aesthetic (Cosmetic) Plastic Surgery (in Toronto in 1994) that the average size of the erect penis is smaller than we have been led to believe.

Two methods of treatment appear to have some merit. The most significant changes have been achieved by a lengthening operation first developed in China and brought to Canada a few years ago. The most relevant anatomical detail is that the structures which make up the penis are partly outside the rest of the body as the penis' shaft, but continue inside for a considerable distance.

The procedure of lengthening the penis is really two stages, the actual operation, and most important, the post-surgical therapy. The operation involves making an incision above and at the base of the penis, releasing the strong fibres which attach the base of the penis to the bone, and filling the resulting space by shifting some muscle from the area next to the penis prior to closure of the incision. However, this only sets the stage for the very important phase of therapy which goes on for many weeks after surgery. This involves wrapping the penis shaft with a bandage to which are attached small weights, usually like those used to balance automobile wheels, which are gradually increased. The weights are worn continuously, and success of the procedure is very dependent on their use.

Through the use of this method, some impressive results in length increase have been achieved, which some men with very small penises getting normal or near normal size. From beginnings with men with obviously very small penises, Dr. Stubbs and surgeons he has trained, have also done the procedure on men with more normal size, who for other reasons desire enlargements.

Other methods which have been used are similar to the methods I favour for lip enlargement, dermis-fat grafting and fat injections. (see Lip Enlargement chapter)The main aim of these is to increase bulk. The injection of fat, as explained elsewhere, has the advantage of being simple but the disadvantage of likely being less lasting than other methods. Dermis fat grafting, on the other hand, may be longer lasting but has a slightly higher risk of infection and involves more surgery.

Plastic surgeons have been understandibly cautious about adding penis enlargement to their practices. Male patients are, in general, more likely to become angry, depressed, agitated, or even suicidal, if they are dissatisfied with the results of their surgery, and sometimes severe psychotic breakdown occurs even when the surgery has resulted in a dramatic improvement. In the past, surgery on the adult male nose was the most likely to result in severe psychiatric problems. Operating on the male genitals would seem to be many times riskier, and the early experience has shown that these patients require a tremendous degree of pre- and post-surgical support. It seems that for carefully selected patients, however, the surgery can be very successful. However, the surgery is still relatively new, and the long-term results still need evaluation.

APPENDIX

FREQUENTLY ASKED QUESTIONS

A. GENERAL

Will it hurt?

During surgery, anaesthesia ensures that you are comfort-able and feel little or no pain. If general anaesthesia is used, you will sleep through the entire operation. After surgery, pain or discomfort is usually mild, and can be controlled with mild pain medication and will usually subside within a few days. Most patients take prescription pain medications for only a few days after surgery.

Is it safe?

Millions of cosmetic plastic surgery operations are done every year and complications are uncommon. But it is not like a visit to a hair stylist. No matter how simple or safe today's cosmetic plastic surgery may seem you must remember that it is still surgery, and as with any surgery, there are risks.

Is it expensive?

Not really. Surgical fees have gone up slowly over the years, and now, with most surgery being done in day surgery clinics, the facility costs are very moderate, compared to hospital costs.

Will there be scars?

All surgery requiring incisions results in scars. However, plastic surgeons are skilled at making incisions so the resulting scars will be as short as possible and will blend into the natural creases and folds of the skin. If newer, endoscopic techniques can be used, the scars will be very small. Most scars will fade over time and become barely noticeable.

Am I a suitable patient for cosmetic surgery?

If you have something definite about your appearance which you would like to have changed, and a plastic surgeon feels there is a good probability of achieving what you desire; if your emotional status is reasonably stable; if you are aware of the risks; and if your general health is good, then you are probably a suitable person to undergo surgery.

I don't want to look strange, or "plastic". How can I prevent that?

The most natural looking results are the best. Good plastic surgery often goes unnoticed. It should improve your appearance without drawing attention to itself. If current techniques are used and you do not make unreasonable and extreme requests, most surgery results in changes which do not appear fake, or unnatural.

Will it hurt?

Of course the degree of discomfort varies from one operation to another and every patient perceives and responds to pain differently. However, it is rare for powerful pain medications to be required.

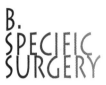

B.
SPECIFIC
SURGERY

1. REJUVENATIVE FACIAL SURGERY

What is the right age to have surgery?

The right age to have surgery is when you feel you have sufficient appearance of aging to be willing to undergo a significant surgical operation, its risks, and the necessary recovery period; when the surgeon feels significant benefit would be achieved from the operation, and when your general health is good.

For a facelift this may be at the age of forty, fifty, sixty, or into the seventies. Doing the operation early to make it "more effective" seems to me to be a way of selling the operation to patients before they are ready. It is rare for me to consider a facelift on a patient less than the early forties. There seem to be two peak age groups: the early to mid-forties, and from fifty through the mid-sixties, although I have done facelifts on patients in their late seventies.

In young patients with familial bulging of the fat in the lower eyelids, surgery can be well worthwhile, even in the mid-twenties. Many patients finally come to have the surgery in their thirties and forties and have had the same appearance of their lower lids since their teens.

Brow lifts, similarly, should be done when the time is right. If there are deep vertical frown lines, they can be treated by muscle reduction whenever present, since drooping of the brows is not uncommon by the mid-thirties.

There is no evidence that doing a "mini-facelift" early makes the face age better, but many patients begin to benefit from current techniques by the early 40's. However excellent results may be achieved at any age from the forties through the seventies, when and if the patient feels it is time.

What is the recovery time?

I usually tell my facelift patients to plan on ten working days away from work, but for younger, healthy patients to return to work in a week is not unusual. The recovery from endoscopic forehead lifts and eyelid surgery is often faster, and return to work in a week is the rule rather than the exception.

Full recovery is, however, incomplete at these times. Healing goes on long beyond the removal of stitches. Scars become thicker and redder during the first few weeks, and then gradually fade. This process takes many weeks and final settling of scars to a soft, flat, pale appearance may take up to a year or longer.

Will there be bruising?

Surgery always involves some form of incision and work beneath the surface, and this means some small veins and arteries must be cut. Surgeons use devices to seal off any significant blood vessels but the tiniest vessels, and capillaries seal better if your own body clotting system is allowed to do the work. For this reason, anything which impairs this function, such as the use of aspirin and other anti-inflammatories, Vitamin E, and some homeopathic remedies must be avoided. If you bruise or bleed easily, you must tell your surgeon in advance, because there may be a problem with your ability to clot, and certain tests may be justified to look for bleeding problems.

However, bruising is usually not very extensive, although it varies greatly from one patient to another.

What about the laser?

Lasers have certain well-defined benefits in cosmetic surgery (see Laser Resurfacing chapter) but the use of the cutting laser as a surgical scalpel seems to be of more benefit in selling an operation than it is to the patient. Studies have shown that there is no benefit in terms of bleeding, bruising, healing time, or to the final result.

How long will the results last?

The typical response to this question has been that surgery does not stop the "clock", it merely sets back the time on the clock of aging. This answer, while a good one, is incomplete. Using current facelift methods, some of the changes are profound and long lasting, such as the removal of fat from the neck and re-alignment of neck muscles, and the removal of bulging fat and excess skin from the eyelids, while other areas follow the "setting the clock back" analogy more closely.

Will I look "pulled" or "tight"?

Not if current techniques are used appropriately

2. COSMETIC NOSE SURGERY

At what age can a nose be treated?

It is usually safe to operate when the facial bones have stopped growing, which in girls is between fourteen and sixteen and in boys is usually between sixteen and eighteen and, of course, when the patient is emotionally mature enough for the procedure.

Will I get a lot of bruising?

This depends partly on your own response to surgery, but mainly on how much bone work must be done.

Will you have to break the bones?

This depends on the shape of your own nose. We do not break; we cut the bone, and this is necessary for several reasons, including as part of straightening the nose, to narrow a wide nose, and to bring the bones together after a large bump has been removed from the bridge.

3. SUCTION LIPOPLASTY

Will the fat come back?

Because the thickness of the "fat organ" is reduced in the areas treated, the changes are permanent. Excess food intake will, as before, result in fat accumulation, but this will occur more in other, untreated parts of the body.

How long do I need to wear the garment or girdle?

I usually recommend three to six weeks, depending on the degree of skin looseness, the age of the patient, and the amount of fat removed, and I examine the patient several times during the healing period. Often, the garment can be removed for periods and bicycle shorts, or similar elasticized garments, can be substituted.

When can I resume exercise?

I encourage walking during the first few days after surgery, light aerobic exercise (treadmill or stationary bicycle) ten to fourteen days after surgery, and full activity after three weeks. Swimming is also fine, and can be started quite early.

4. BODY CONTOUR SURGERY

Should I wait to have a "tummy tuck" until I have had all my children?

In general, if you are planning to have more children, some of the benefits may be lost. However, if you have lost weight and have excess skin as a result, or feel self conscious about your appearance, the results of surgery may justify the operation at any time.

Won't liposuction take care of it?

When there is skin looseness and the underlying muscles

are stretched, suction will not improve the appearance and may worsen it. When there is significant fat and some skin looseness, suction may not give a predictable result. In some cases, it is reasonable to start with a preliminary suction operation, with the understanding that a secondary (tightening) body contour surgery may be needed.

Do I need to have such a long scar?

The incision length depends mostly on how wide an area of skin is removed, and this is related to how loose the skin is. In an abdominoplasty (tummy tuck), when all the skin below the belly button is removed, the scar usually runs from hip to hip. Less looseness requires a smaller incision.

When can I start exercising again?

I encourage walking during the first few days, light aerobic activity at two weeks, and full exercise routine with abdominal exercises at six weeks.

5. BREAST AUGMENTATION

For the answers to most questions relating to breast augmentation, consult the chapter entitled "Breast Augmentation"

Are these new, saline implants, safe?

Saline implants are not new. They were also used from the early 1960's, but were used less frequently than silicone gel implants. In general, the implants have a very good long term safety record, but an extensive explanation to discuss the many specific concerns you may have is found in the chapter on breast augmentation.

Do I need to have them changed every five years?

Although the implants can leak, collapsing in the process, and allowing the saline to escape, this is an uncommon event, especially in the first five years. When leaks occur, deflation is quite rapid, and harmless. Removal of the implant and replacement is generally a simple procedure, so periodic replacement before leakage occurs does not seem to be worthwhile.

Can I fly in an airplane or SCUBA dive?

Yes. There is no change in the pressure within the implant at altitude or underwater, so there is no increased risk of rupture.

6. BREAST UPLIFT

Should I have this done if I am planning to have more children?

This depends on how much smaller your breasts are than prior to your first pregnancy, and how much distress the shape of your breasts causes you. If you have lost a lot of breast volume, an augmentation with lift will give you significant improvement, and might only require a smaller secondary tightening if you become pregnant and lose some of your shape again.

Will I lose feeling?

Most of the time, changes in feeling are mild. Numbness, or even excess sensitivity are possible, but usually improve with time

Is breast feeding possible?

The function of the breast is not usually changed by lift surgery.

Office "intake sheet",
for medical history information

BENJAMIN GELFANT M D FRCSC
Suite 902 805 West Broadway
Vancouver, B. C. V5Z 1K1

NAME _____ AGE _____ DATE _____

REQUESTING INFORMATION REGARDING : _____

WERE YOU REFERRED BY:
Family member ❑ friend ❑ family doctor ❑ specialist ❑ yellow pages ❑ other ❑

	YES	NO
Have you had surgery before?	❑	❑

If yes, please list operations:_____

| Have you had any problems with general anaesthesia? | ❑ | ❑ |
| Family history of anaesthesia problems?malig. hyperthermia | ❑ | ❑ |

List any regular medications _____

List any allergies _____ allergic to latex?

Do you bruise easily or bleed excessively?	❑	❑
Do you drink alcohol;	❑	❑
Do you smoke? yes q no q In the past?	❑	❑
Is there a chance you are pregnant?	❑	❑
Do you have any dental crowns or bridges	❑	❑
Do you take aspirin or anti-inflammatories	❑	❑

Have you ever had any of the following? :

ULCER/HIATUS HERNIA/INDIGESTION	❑	KIDNEY, LIVER DISEASE	❑
BLOOD CLOTS	❑	TRANSFUSION?	❑
BRONCHITIS/ASTHMA//EMPHYSEMA	❑	ANEMIA	❑
SHORTNESS OF BREATH	❑	THYROID DISEASE	❑
HEART CONDITION	❑	DIABETES	❑
HIGH BLOOD PRESSURE	❑	CORTISONE TREATMENT	❑
RHEUM. FEVER/HEART VALVE DISEASE	❑	ARTHRITIS	❑
HEART MURMUR	❑	EPILEPSY	❑
CHEST PAIN/ANGINA/ PALPITATIONS	❑	HEADACHES	❑
PACEMAKER	❑	GLAUCOMA	❑
STROKE/DIZZINESS	❑	BACK PROBLEMS	❑

Surgery request form
(Example: individualized for each type of procedure)

REQUEST FOR SURGERY - SUCTION LIPOPLASTY (FAT SUCTION)

(AREAS) _____ Date _____ Time _____

1. I, _____ , authorize   BENJAMIN GELFANT, MD
and his/her associates to perform surgery for _____
                                                          (Myself or Minor)

2. I am aware that the practice of medicine and surgery is not an exact science, and I acknowledge that no guarantes have been made to me as to the results of the operation or procedure.

3. The procedure listed above has been explained to me and I understand that there may be complications including but not limited to the following:

   a. permanent scars will result from this surgery. In some cases the scars will become thickened and/oror wide;
   b. the procedure is subject to the same possible complications as all other surgical procedures, such as infection, bleeding or failure to heal, which would require appropriate treatment including possible further surgery;
   c. sensation can be altered temporarily or permanently;
   d. alterations in circulation can occur which could result in loss in skin;
   e. in some cases secondary procedures will be necessary to improve the final result;
   f. symmetry is not always achieved;
   g. bleeding can occur which could require blood transfusions with their inherent risks;
   h. skin irregularities, lumpiness, hardness, or dimpling may occur which could be permanent;
   i. loose saggy skin can result from this procedure necessitating further surgery with longer incisions to remove the excess skin;
   j. areas of "cellulite" will be changed little or not at all by this procedure;

4. I recognize that, during the course of the operation, unforeseen conditions may necessitate additional or different procedures than those set forth above. I therefore further authorize and request that the above named surgeon, his/her assistants, or designees perform such procedures as are, in his/her professional judgment, necessary and desirable, including, but not limited to, procedures involving pathology and radiology. The authority granted under Paragraph 4 shall extend to remedying conditions that are not known to the above doctors at the time of the operation is commenced.

5. I consent to the administration of anaesthesia, with the exception of _____ to be given by the above doctors or such anaesthesiologists as they shall select. I understand that adverse reactions to anaesthetic drugs can occur.

6. I am allergic to the following medicines; _____

7. I consent to be photographed before, during, and after the treatment. These photographs shall be the property of the above doctors and may be published in scientific journals and/or shown for scientific reasons.

8. I agree to keep the above doctors informed of any change of address so that they can notify me of any late findings, and I agree to cooperate with the above doctors in my care after surgery until completely discharged.

9. I have read the above request and fully understand it. I acknowledge that I have been advised as to the alternative methods of treatment, have been given an opportunity to ask all questions regarding the treatment to be administered, and am satisfied that I have been fully informed and understand the procedure.

Witness_____Patient_____

Pre-op instructions
(Example: individualized
for each procedure)

SUCTION LIPOPLASTY INSTRUCTIONS

BEFORE YOUR SURGERY

1. No aspirin (ASA) or medicine containing aspirin-like products* for 2 weeks before surgery, since they interfere with normal blood clotting. *Check the list at the end of these instructions and if in doubt, call us.If needed, ,Acetaminophen (Tylenol) instead.
No vitamin E for 2 weeks prior to surgery.

2. Smokers should cut down to no more than 3 or 4 cigarettes a day for 3 days before surgery to reduce postoperative coughing and possible bleeding.

3. Report any signs of a cold, infection, boils or pustules appearing 3 weeks before surgery.

4. Arrange for someone to drive you to your home, hotel or motel after surgery.

DAY OF SURGERY

Arrive at_____ hrs.

Address:_____

1. Nothing to eat or drink after midnight the night before.

2. Do not take medication of any kind (unless instructed by Dr. Gelfant). Your preoperative medications will be given to you upon arrival.

3. Wear comfortable, loose fitting clothes which do not have to be put over head. No pantihose, please.

4. You must have someone to drive for you after surgery.

On arrival at the office, give secretary your driver's name and phone number, as well as address and phone number where you will be the night after surgery.

5. You must have someone spend the first day and night with you. If you do not have this available, please tell us and we will make other arrangements for you. Additional instructions can be given to the person calling for you.

6. If you have any questions before your operation, please call our office weekdays between 9:00 a.m. and 5:00 p.m.

AFTER YOUR OPERATION

1. Take medications according to instructions on bottle. If taking narcotics, or if other pain medications make you feel "spacey" or drowsy, have someone else give you your medicines according to the proper time intervals. Under such circumstances, you could forget and take them too often.

2. Rest in bed for the first 24 hours. You may get up to go to the bathroom or for short walks with help. After the first day, go for frequent short walks.

3. Begin taking an iron supplement with a multivitamin.

4. You may return to work in 3-4 days, avoiding strenuous activity or heavy lifting. It may cause you to bleed.

5. You are required to wear a compression garment for the first four post-operative days without removing it for any purpose. During this time, you are allowed to shower (have someone assist you the first day in case of a fainting spell), drying the garment with a towel and hair dryer.

6. The garment may be removed for bathing and washing of the garment after the first 4 days. Otherwise, wear continuously during daily activities for the next 4 w e e k s . You may replace the compression garment with a pair of snug fitting bike or exercise pants for comfort.

7. Avoid smoking for 48 hours after your operation to prevent coughing and   possible bleeding.

8. No alcohol for 5 days post-operatively.

9. You can expect:
>   (a) Moderate discomfort - use pain medication and/or cool compresses
>   (b) Moderate swelling
>   (c) Large amount of black and blue discoloration
>   (d) Some bleeding from incisions

10. Call 874-2078 if you have:
>   (a) Severe pain not responding to medications
>   (b) Marked swelling, or obviously more swelling on one side than the other.
>   (c) If any other questions or problem arises

11. You may read or watch television.

12. Avoid prolonged exposure to sun and heat for one month to avoid swelling.

13. Feel free to call upon us at any time. We want you to be as comfortable as possible during your healing period.

OFFICE VISITS: 1st: 2 to 3 days following surgery
                2nd: 1 week to 10 days

*ASA or anti-inflammatory containing drugs

Anacin, ASA, Bufferin, Calmine,Coricidin, Coryphen, Dolomine,Dristan Capsules, Entrophen, Herbopyrine, Instantine, Kalmex, Madelon, MED Tigol, Midol, Nervine, Nezger Norgesic, Novasen, Novo AC&C, Pain AID, Robaxisal, 217, 222, 282, 292's, Upsarin. Also AC with codeine, Asantine, Coryphen, Darvon products, Endodan, Fiorinal, Novopropoxyn, Oxycodan, Painex, Percodan, Phenaphen, Robaxisal, 692, Tecnal, 282's, 292's,Artrol, Trilisate, Diclofenac (Apo-Diclo, Apo-Diclo SR, Arthrotec, Diclofenac Ect, Novo-Difenac, Novo-Difenac SR, Nu-Diclo, Taro-Diclofenac, Voltaren, Voltaren SR), Diclofenac potassium (Voltaren Rapide), Diflunisal (Apo-Diflunisal, Dolobid, Novo-Diflunisal, Nu-Diflunisal), Etodolac (Ultradol), Fenoprofen calcium (Nalfon), Floctafenine (Idarac), Flurbiprofen (Ansaid, Apo-Flurbiprofen FC, Froben, Froben SR, Novo-Flurprofen,Nu-Flurbiprofen), Ibuprofen

(Actiprofen, Advil, Advil Cold & Sinus, Amersol, Apo-Ibuprofen, Excedrin IB, Medipren, Motrin, Motrin IB, Novo-Profen, Nuprin, Nu-Ibuprofen, Sinus Pr & Pain Reliever with Ibuprofen), Indomethacin (Apo-Indomethacin, Indocid, Indocid SR, Indolec, Novo-Methacin, Nu-Indo, Pro-Indo, Rhodacine), Ketroprofen (Apo-Keto, Apo-Keto-E, Novo-Keto, Novo-Keto-Ec, Nu-Ketroprofen, Nu-Ketroprofen-E, Orudis, Orudis E, Orudis SR, Oruvail, PMS-Ketoprofen, PMS-Ketroprofen-E,Rhodis, Rhodis-EC), Ketorolac tromethamine (Acular, Toradol), Magnesium salicylate (Back-Ese-M, Doan's Backache Pills, Herbogesic), Mefenamic acid (Ponstan), Nabumetone (Relafen), Naproxen (Apo-Naproxen, Naprosyn, Naprosyn-E, Naxen, Novo-Naprox, Nu-Naprox, PMS-Naproxen), Naproxen sodium, anaprox, anaprox DS, Apo-Napro-Na, Naproxin-Na, Novo-Naprox Sodium, Synflex, Synflex DS, Oxyphenbutazone, Oxybutazone, Phenylbutazone, Alka Phenyl, Alka Phenylbutazone, Apo-Phenylbutazone, Butazolidin, Novo-Butazone, Phenylone Plus, Piroxicam, Apo-Piroxicam, Feldene, Kenral-Piroxican, Novo-Pirocam, Nu-Pirox, PMS-Piroxicam, Pro-Piroxicam, Rho-Piroxicam, Salsalate, Disalcid, Sodium Salicylate, Dodd's, Dodd's Extra-Strength, Sulindac, Apo-Sulin, Clinoril, Novo-Sundac, Nu-Sulindac, Sulindac, Tenoxicam, Mobilflex, Tiaprofenic acid, Albert Tiafen, Apo-Tiaprofenic, Surgam, Surgam SR, Tolmetin sodium, Novo-Tolmetin, Tolectin

GLOSSARY

Abdominoplasty ("Tummy Tuck")
16,829 performed by board-certified plastic surgeons in 1994*
Sometimes after multiple pregnancies or large weight loss, abdominal muscles weaken, and skin in the area becomes loose. Abdominoplasty can tighten the skin and abdominal muscles and remove some stretch marks. In both men and women, the procedure will remove excess skin and fat. Generally, an incision is made across the pubic area and around the umbilicus (navel). When skin laxity and muscle weakness is confined to the lower part of the abdomen, a modified abdominoplasty that limits tissue removal and muscle repair to the area below the umbilicus may be performed. This usually leaves a shorter scar and no scarring around the navel.

Alpha Hydroxy Acids
Alpha hydroxy acids are derived from foods such as fruits and milk, and can improve the texture of skin by removing layers of dead cells and encouraging cell regeneration.

Arm Lift (Brachioplasty)
Excess fat in the upper arms can sometimes be reduced through liposuction alone or may require skin excision as well if there is loose, drooping skin.

Augmentation Mammoplasty (see Breast Augmentation)

Blepharoplasty (see Eyelid Surgery)

Brachioplasty (see Arm Lift)

Breast Augmentation (Augmentation Mammoplasty)

39,247 performed by board-certified plastic surgeons in 1994*

Breast augmentation is typically performed to enlarge small breasts, underdeveloped breasts or breasts that have decreased in size after a woman has had children. It is accomplished by surgically inserting an implant behind each breast. An incision is made either under the breast, around the areola (the pink skin surrounding the nipple) or in the armpit. A pocket is created for the implant either behind the breast tissue or behind the muscle between the breast and the chest wall.

Breast Lift (Mastopexy)

10,053 performed by board-certified plastic surgeons in 1994*

Frequently, a woman elects this surgery after losing a considerable amount of weight, or losing volume and tone in her breasts after having children. The plastic surgeon relocates the nipple and areola (the pink skin surrounding the nipple) to a higher position, repositions the breast tissue to a higher level, removes excess skin from the lower portion of the breast and then reshapes the remaining breast skin. Scars are around the areola, extending vertically down the breast and horizontally along the crease underneath the breast. Variations on this technique, in some cases, may result in less noticeable scarring.

Breast Reduction (Reduction Mammoplasty)

36,074 performed by board-certified plastic surgeons in 1994*

Breast reduction is normally classified as a reconstructive procedure, since oversize breasts interfere with normal function and physical activity. However, there is an important aesthetic component to the operation, since the plastic surgeon can improve the shape of the breasts and nipple areas.

Breast reduction involves removing excess breast tissue and skin, repositioning the nipple and areola (the pink skin surrounding the nipple) and reshaping the remaining breast tissue.

Buccal Fat Pad

Buccal fat pads are located above the jawline near the corner of the mouth. They can be removed in individuals with excessively round faces to give a more contoured look, sometimes referred to as the "waif look." However, plastic surgeons warn that, in some individuals, removal of the buccal fat pads can lead to a drawn, hollow-cheeked look as aging progresses.

Buttock Lift

Excess fat and loose skin in the buttock area can be reduced by performing a buttock lift in combination with liposuction. Incisions required for skin removal can often be hidden within bathing suit lines

Buffered Phenol Peel

Buffered phenol offers an option for severely sun-damaged skin. One such formula uses olive oil, among other ingredients, to diminish the strength of the phenol solution. Another slightly milder formula uses glycerin. Buffered phenol peels may be more comfortable for patients, and the skin heals faster than with a standard phenol peel.

Calf Augmentation

Increased fullness of the calf can be achieved using implants made of firm silicone which are inserted from behind the knee and moved into position underneath the calf muscle.

Cannula

A hollow tube attached to a high-vacuum device used to remove fat through liposuction. The plastic surgeon manipulates the cannula within the fat layers under the skin, dislodging the fat and "vacuuming" it out.

Capsular Contracture

Capsular contracture is the most common problem associated with breast implants. It occurs when naturally forming scar tissue around the implant shrinks and tightens, making the breast feel firmer than normal and sometimes causing pain and an unnatural appearance of the breast. Capsular contracture is not a health concern, but moderate to severe contracture can make mammography more difficult.

Chemical Peel

Fine lines and wrinkles around the mouth and on the forehead and cheek areas may be improved with a wide range of skin treatments. A chemical peel solution is applied to the entire face or to specific areas to peel away the skin's top layers. Several light to medium-depth peels can often achieve similar results to one deeper peel treatment, with less risk and shorter recovery time. Peel solutions may contain alpha hydroxy acids, tricholoracetic acid (TCA) or phenol as the peeling agent, depending on the depth of peel desired and on other patient selection factors.

Cellulite

Cellulite is the dimpled-looking fat that often appears on the buttocks, thighs and hips. While there is no treatment that will eradicate this problem, aesthetic plastic surgeons are exploring techniques which may improve the condition. One method is to cut the fibrous tissue that binds the fat down in these areas and creates the lumpy appearance, and then to inject fact withdrawn from elsewhere in the body to smooth out the unevenness. Another technique, called the cellulite lift, surgically removes excess skin and fat, leaving a thin scar that may extend around the full circumference of the abdomen but is placed discreetly within bikini lines.

Chin Augmentation (Mentoplasty)

3,632 performed by board-certified plastic surgeons in 1994*

Chin augmentation can strengthen the appearance of a receding chin by increasing its projection. The procedure does not affect the patient's bite or jaw. There are two techniques. One is performed through an incision inside the mouth and involves moving the chinbone, then wiring it into position.The other approach requires insertion of an implant through an incision under the chin.

Collagen Injections

Collagen is an injectable protein obtained from the deeper layers of cow skin that can be used to treat facial wrinkles. Patients to be treated with collagen should first be tested for any allergic reaction. The results of collagen injections are not permanent, and treatments must be repeated periodically to maintain results.

Cosmetic Tattooing

Cosmetic tattooing, or micropigmentation, can be used for permanent eyeliner, eyebrows or lip color. It can also be used for permanent blush and eyeshadow, though this is infrequent. Other uses by plastic surgeons include recreating the coloration of the areola around the nipple following breast reconstruction; restoring the color of dark or light skin where natural pigmentation has been lost through such factors as vitiligo, cancer, burns or other scarring; and eliminating some types of birthmarks or previous tattoos. Micropigmentation should be performed only under medical supervision by appropriately trained personnel.

Dermabrasion

Dermabrasion is a procedure in which a high-speed rotary wheel, similar to fine-grained sandpaper, is used to abrade the skin. It may be recommended when there is extensive sun damage and heavy skin wrinkling. In addition, dermabrasion can be used to improve the texture of pockmarked skin resulting from severe acne or chicken pox. Following treatment, the skin should appear firmer and smoother, but permanent pigment changes may occur. Dermabrasion is done less frequently today, since the advent of pulsed lasers.

Earlobe Reduction

A simple, 30-minute procedure, earlobe reduction can be performed in a plastic surgeon's office or at the same time as a facelift operation. When the lobe appears disproportionately long, a wedge is removed, the edges brought together and repaired.

Eyelid Surgery (Blepharoplasty)

50,838 performed by board-certified plastic surgeons in 1994*

Aesthetic eyelid surgery can brighten the face and restore a more youthful appearance by reducing the fat that causes bags beneath the eyes and removing wrinkled, drooping layers of skin on the eyelids. Blepharoplasty is often performed along with a facelift or with other facial rejuvenation procedures. Incisions follow the natural contour lines in both upper and lower lids, or can be done through the lining of the lower eyelid, providing access to skin and fatty tissue. The thin surgical scars are usually barely visible and blend into the eye's natural lines and folds.

Facelift (Rhytidectomy)

32,283 performed by board-certified plastic surgeons in 1994*

A facelift can reduce sagging skin and deeper soft structures on the face and neck. Incisions are placed so as to be concealed as much as possible; the exact design of incisions may vary from patient to patient and according to the surgeon's personal technique. When necessary, removal of fatty deposits beneath the skin and tightening of sagging muscles is performed. The slack in the skin itself is then taken up and the excess removed. Scars can usually be concealed by makeup.

Fat Injections

Fat withdrawn from one body site can be injected into another - for example, to smooth lines in the face or build up other features such as the lips. Fat injection is still not widely performed by plastic surgeons, primarily because of skepticism about the longevity of results. In most cases, a large percentage of injected fat is resorbed by the body, and the procedure must be repeated periodically to maintain results. Injection of fat to enlarge the breasts is not recommended because of the possibility of dense scarring that may seriously hinder accurate interpretation of both breast self-exams and mammograms.

Forehead Lift (Brow Lift)
13,182 performed by board-certified plastic surgeons in 1994*

The forehead lift is designed to correct or improve skin wrinkling, as well as loss of tone and sagging of the eyebrows that often occurs as part of the aging process. The procedure may also help to smooth horizontal expression lines in the forehead and vertical frown lines between the eyebrows. The procedure may now be performed with the use of an endoscope, requiring much shorter incisions. Improvements are made beneath the skin and on the deep muscles; skin and muscle are then tightened to give a fresher, more youthful appearance.

Hydroxyapatite Granules

Hydroxyapatite granules are a bone substitute made from coral that can be used to enhance facial contours, such as forming more prominent cheekbones. The substance also has reconstructive uses in craniofacial surgery.

Lasers

The past few years have seen dramatic advances in the use of lasers for resurfacing, or rejuvenating sun, age and environmentally damaged skin. Lasers can be effectively used to eliminate surface blood vessels on the face that become reddened and enlarged due to sun exposure. Lasers are being used by some surgeons for eyelid surgery and facelifts, but the benefits have not been proven and risks may be increased.

Lip Augmentation

One of the most effective methods of augmenting the lips is surgically advancing the lip forward, with incisions placed inside the mouth. A dermal-fat graft, taken from the deeper layers of the skin, may then be positioned under the mucosa (the lining of the lip) to add additional "plumpness". Injecting fat for lip augmentation is still an alternative, but the correction is not permanent, and injections must be repeated periodically to maintain results.

Lip Reduction
To reduce the lips, a small strip of the mucosa (the lining of the lip) is surgically removed to narrow the lips to the desired proportion. The small scars on the outside of the lips are barely noticeable.

Suction Lipoplasty (Liposuction)
51,072 performed by board-certified plastic surgeons in 1994*
Liposuction allows the plastic surgeon to remove localized collections of fatty tissue from the legs, buttocks, abdomen, back, arms, face and neck using a vacuum device. The procedure leaves only short scars, one-half inch in length or less. The use of refined equipment allows removal from delicate areas such as calves and ankles. Liposuction removes fat, but it cannot eliminate dimpling or correct skin laxity. If a patient's skin has lost much of its elasticity, the plastic surgeon may recommend a skin tightening procedure such as a thigh lift, buttock lift or arm lift, all of which leave more extensive scars.

Malar (Cheekbone) Augmentation
The cheekbones may be built up by placing an implant over them. This is usually performed through an incision within the mouth, but it may be done through a lower eyelid or brow lift incision.

Mastopexy (see Breast Lift)

Otoplasty (Ear Surgery)
The ears are positioned closer to the head by reshaping the cartilage (supporting tissue). This is usually accomplished through incisions placed behind the ears so that subsequent scars will be concealed in a natural skin crease. Otoplasty can be performed on children as early as age five or six.

Phenol
The chemical phenol is sometimes used for full-face peeling when sun damage or wrinkling is severe. It can also be used to treat limited areas of the face, such as deep wrinkles around the mouth, but it may permanently

bleach the skin, leaving a line of demarcation between the treated and untreated areas that must be covered with makeup. This is much less commonly done today because lasers have largely supplanted peels.

Platysma
The muscle which, when tight and firm, gives the neck underneath the chin and jawline its youthful contour. The platysma muscle can be tightened during a facelift or as a separate procedure.

Reduction Mammoplasty (see Breast Reduction)

Retin-A
Retin-A cream or lotion may be applied to enhance the overall texture of the skin and is often prescribed as a pre-treatment prior to a facelift, chemical peel, or laser resurfacing.

Rhinoplasty (Nose Reshaping)
35,927 performed by board-certified plastic surgeons in 1994*

Rhinoplasty is usually performed to alter the size and shape of the bridge and tip of the nose. Reshaping is generally done through incisions inside the nose, often with and incision passing across the central portion of the nose between the nostrils. It is sometimes necessary to narrow the base of the nose or reduce the size of the nostrils, which involves removing small wedges of skin at the base of the nostrils. The nose is reduced, or sometimes built up, by adjusting its bone and cartilage, the supporting structures. The skin and soft tissues then redrape themselves over this new "scaffolding ".

Rhytidectomy (see Facelift)

SMAS
The superficial musculoaponeurotic system (SMAS) is a layer of tissue that covers the deeper structures in the cheek area and is in continuity with the superficial muscle covering the lower face and neck, called the platysma.

Most facelifts today lift and reposition the SMAS as well as the skin.

Superficial and Syringe Liposculpture
Use of a syringe to withdraw fat, instead of vacuum suctioning pumps, allows for less blood loss and speedier postoperative recovery. Superficial syringe, liposculpture is performed on the layer of fat just beneath the skin.

TCA
Trichloroacetic acid is used for peeling of the face, neck, hands and other exposed areas of the body. It has less bleaching effect than phenol, and is excellent for "spot" peeling of specific areas. It can be used for deep, medium or light peeling, depending on the concentration and method of
application.

Textured-Surface Breast Implants
The shell of textured-surface breast implants are made with the same silicone elastomer that is used for the shell of other types of breast implants, but a special manufacturing process creates a textured surface. Some studies have suggested that the textured surface may help to reduce the incidence of capsular contracture, tightening of the naturally forming scar tissue around the implant which can make the breast feel firmer than normal.

Thigh Lift
A thigh lift can be performed to tighten sagging skin in the thigh area. Outer thigh lifts are combined with buttock lifts, with incisions following the bikini lines around the waist. Inner thigh lifts lift the inner upper thigh. They may be combined in a "lower body lift" and used with or without preliminary suction lipoplasty.

Tissue expansion
Tissue expansion is a technique in which skin or other tissue is stretched using inflatable balloons. It can be of particular value in performing breast reconstruction, breast enlargement or treatment of male pattern baldness.

Transconjunctival blepharoplasty

Transconjunctival blepharoplasty (eyelid surgery) is performed by making an incision inside the lower eyelid. It avoids any scarring on the lower lid and may reduce the possibility of the eyelid pulling down, which may occur as a postoperative complication in some patients. It is a useful technique when only fat, and not skin or muscle, needs to be removed from the eyelid area.

Source for plastic surgery statistics: American Society of Plastic and Reconstructive Surgeons

APPROXIMATE FEES

The following gives you a current idea of what surgery will cost. Fees listed include all costs, including surgical fees, anaesthesia, operating room or ambulatory clinic charges, and taxes, where applicable.

Consultation	$80-$150
Facelift	$5,000-$8,500
Face & Forehead Lift	$10,000-$12,000
Forehead Lift (endoscopic)	$3,500-$4,500
Upper & Lower Eyelids	$2,500-$3,500
Upper or Lower Eyelids	$1,500-$2,500
Laser Resurfacing:	
(a) small area	$1,200-$2,000
(b) full face	$2,500-$5,000
Rhinoplasty (nose)	$2,000-$5,000
Liposuction	$2,000-$6,000 & up
Breast Augmentation	$4,500-$6,000
Breast Uplift	$3,000-$5,500
Breast Uplift with Augmentation	$6,000+
Abdominoplasty (tummy tuck)	$5,000-$7,500
Thigh lift	$6,000-$12,000

Further Reading

Bordo, Susan
Unbearable Weight. Feminism, Western Culture, and the Body
Berkeley: University of California Press, 1993.

Freedman, Rita
Beauty Bound
Lexington, Mass.: Lexington Books, 1986.

Friday, Nancy
The Power of Beauty
New York: Harper Collins, 1996.

Hatfield, Elaine and Sprecher, Susan
Mirror . . .the Importance of Looks in Everyday Life
Albany: State University of New York Press, 1986.

Wilson, Josleen
The American Society of Plastic & Reconstructive Surgeons:
Guide to Cosmetic Surgery
Simon & Suster, 1992

For Further Information:

Canadian Society for Aesthetic(Cosmetic) Plastic Surgery
1-416-831-7750

American Society for Plastic and Reconstructive Surgery
1-800-635-0635
http://www.plasticsurgery.org

American Society for Aesthetic Surgery
1-888-2727711
http://surgery.org

Benjamin Gelfant MD FRCSC Inc.
1-604-874-2078
http://dr-ben-plastic-doc.com/